10 98

6 July

the
sleep
solution

the sleep solution

Improve your sleep,
health and quality
of life – from tonight

NIGEL BALL and NICK HOUGH

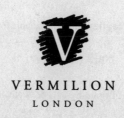

VERMILION
LONDON

3 5 7 9 10 8 6 4 2

Text copyright © Nigel Ball and Nick Hough 1994-1998, 1999

First published in the United Kingdom in 1998 by Vermilion
This new edition published in 1999 by Vermilion

an imprint of Ebury Press
The Random House Group · 20 Vauxhall Bridge Road · London SW1V 2SA

Random House Australia (Pty) Limited
20 Alfred Street · Milsons Point · Sydney · New South Wales 2061 · Australia

Random House New Zealand Limited
18 Poland Road · Glenfield · Auckland 10 · New Zealand

Random House South Africa (Pty) Ltd
Endulini · 5A Jubilee Road · Parktown 2193 · South Africa

The Random House Group Limited Reg. No. 954009
www.randomhouse.co.uk

A CIP catalogue record for this book is available from the British Library

ISBN: 0 09 181971 7

Printed and bound in Great Britain by Cox & Wyman Ltd, Reading, Berkshire.

About the Authors

Nigel Ball and Nick Hough first met in 1976 while working on their doctoral degrees in zoology at Oxford. Since then, Nigel has lived primarily in the United States. Today he is the clinical director of the Sleep Disorders Center at Virginia Mason Medical Center in Seattle. He is also a diplomate of the American Board of Sleep Medicine. His interest in sleep developed out of research he conducted while at Oxford. He is the author of numerous papers, book chapters and articles on sleep. He lives near Seattle with his wife Maggie and their two children, Hazel and Thomas.

In conjunction with his work at Oxford, Nick Hough published a number of scientific papers. After leaving the university, he pursued a totally different career path, entering the world of advertising. He has worked with a number of large agencies in London and Amsterdam and is now the managing director of Leagas Delaney. He lives in London with his wife Ros and their three children, Holly, Lily, and Harry.

Together, Nigel Ball and Nick Hough formed Sleepwell International Limited in 1993. The idea behind this venture is to advise the employees of large corporations on their sleep health. This book – *The Sleep Solution* – came out of that work.

Contents

Acknowledgements

The idea for this book came to us on the Winslow Ferry. We were discussing the horrors of poor sleep, and bemoaning the difficulty that most people experience in getting help. We felt we had to make our knowledge and programme more widely available.

We were fortunate to team up with publishers who not only had progressive ideas about books on positive health but also employ talented, enthusiastic and truly professional people. Our profound thanks to Sarah Sutton, Joanna Carreras, Fiona MacIntyre and Niccy Cowen.

We doubt this book would ever have materialized without our (special) agent Bruce Hyman, who believed in the idea and made sure it came to fruition.

Over the years we have benefited from many fine colleagues. Our time at Oxford together was particularly influential and we cannot hope to express here the depth of each individual's contribution. David McFarland, David Macdonald and Richard Dawkins brought us together and showed us a world of ideas which have influenced us ever since.

Dr Ken Casey, Catherine Darley, Chris Dugmore, Dr Robert Galbraith, Richard Kersh, Dr Steve Kirtland, Dr Joe Leutzinger, Dr Malcolm Newdick, Ken Royall, Dr Jim Shaffery, Dr Ross Sochynsky, Suzanne Stoner, Kay Taylor, and Elliot West are people to whom we wish to express special thanks. Nigel has been lucky to be able to work with two remarkable sleep professionals: Dr Gene Pardee and Dr Doug Schmidt.

Few people are as fortunate with their parents as we have been. Jim Hough was a fine man with a great sense of humour and decency, while Pat Hough first inspired Nick's interest in biology and tolerated all sorts of creepy-crawlies around the house. From the times when Joyce Ball got up at dawn to take Nigel birdwatching, she has always been a wonderful influence. Derek Ball awakened his desire to write and think critically.

Our children, as well as being a constant source of fun and joy, taught us the true value of a good night's sleep. To Hazel, Thomas, Holly, Lily and Harry: may you sleep well and live happily.

Our wives, Ros and Maggie, have been inspirational and tolerant. Few women would have put up with their husbands going out so often to see the Mariners and The Fall, and drinking gallons of Starbucks' coffee and Red Hook under the transparent guise of 'We're working on the book'.

When you should
see your doctor

This is an educational book and programme, and it cannot be a substitute for a comprehensive examination and medical management by your doctor or a qualified sleep specialist. The authors, editors, and publisher of this book have made extensive efforts to ensure that the concepts presented here are accurate and conform to generally accepted clinical and research standards as they exist at the time of publication. However, constant changes in information and knowledge resulting from continual research and clinical experience, reasonable differences of opinion among authorities and the unique aspects of individual clinical situations require that the reader exercise individual judgement when making clinical decisions.

You should definitely see your doctor if:

- you are ever *dangerously* sleepy without an obvious cause (for example, going to work after staying up all night at a party). This includes irresistible sleepiness, accidents or near accidents because you are sleepy.
- you complete this programme and are still frequently sleepy enough for your life to be affected (for example, you are unable to start or complete something that you wanted or needed to do; you miss out on pleasurable activities because you are too sleepy).
- you are worried about your sleep or the things that happen while you are asleep.

Your family doctor can help with medical issues and the common sleep disorders. Sleep specialists deal with the more complex sleep disorders and especially those that do not respond quickly to treatment. They usually work at or with a sleep disorders centre.

Many sleep problems are substantially improved by the small changes that we can make ourselves. Sleep is affected, often subtly, by the way in which sleep and wakefulness are organized. Sleep disorders, general health, and sleep fitness are closely linked, and you can often improve your overall well-being simply by improving your sleep.

Introduction

Only about one in five of us sleeps well with little effort. The rest of us need to work at it. This book will help you to improve the quality of the time you spend asleep in the easiest, most effective and natural way. It will also help you to get more from your sleep, perhaps in ways that you cannot now imagine.

As adults in the modern world, we face many challenges. Responsibilities, the care of children and their after-school activities, late-night television, shift work, commuting and international travel take their toll, making good-quality sleep more important but unfortunately more difficult than ever. As you look around, you'll see tired faces and slumping bodies. Even weekends do not provide the opportunity for catching up on sleep that they used to.

This book offers you practical guidelines to transform the time that you spend asleep. Obviously, if you have trouble sleeping or staying awake, you'll be interested in a sleep programme. But if you feel tired, low, lacking in energy or irritable, the chances are that you also need to pay more attention to your sleep. You may have picked up this book because you're aware that your sleep, or perhaps a family member's sleep, is nowhere near as good as it should be. Is this a problem that has persisted for some time, and you've had little success when you've tried to get help? You may have tried medications and found that each one is effective for a short while and then the problem slowly returns. Or perhaps you can sleep well only when you take a sleeping-pill and you dislike the prospect of a lifetime on that drug. It's not just a question of getting *enough* sleep – your lifestyle, environment, sleep habits, and, most importantly, the quality of your sleep, are also involved.

Many people reading this book will have been dissatisfied with the explanations that have been given for their sleep problems. All too often, serious sleep problems are attributed to stress, hormones, being overweight, or having young children. In this book we have put a lot of effort into providing the tools that will allow you to find a better explanation for your problems, and hence a faster, more effective, solution.

Why do we need to be concerned about getting good-quality sleep?

Poor sleep causes sleepiness which leads to accidents, poor job satisfaction, bad moods, and inadequate social skills. Poor sleep also affects our overall health and survival: our hearts, brains and digestive systems suffer. But the best argument for good sleep health is probably just the joy of waking after a truly refreshing and restorative night's sleep, or feeling energetic and alert all day long. If you can remember those feelings, you will readily understand why it is worth devoting some time and effort to get better sleep.

This book is called *The Sleep Solution*. We chose that title to emphasize not only that there are attainable solutions to sleep problems, but that sleep itself can be a solution to some of life's problems. Sleep can be an important positive influence on our lives.

We believe strongly in the idea that there's more to be done with sleep than just fixing sleep problems. Sleep is a powerful part of our biological heritage that can be used to make our waking time more productive and enjoyable. Sleep fitness is a central idea behind *The Sleep Solution*. This is the concept that anyone – even someone who does not have a sleep disorder – can improve his or her sleep for lasting benefits to health and well-being. With better sleep you'll avoid the problems that result from poor sleep, and also continue to sharpen and brighten your wakefulness. There will be a bonus of a surprisingly large improvement in almost everything that you do.

Sleep fitness is simple:
- Start by recognizing that sleep is an integral part of life itself. No sleep solution will be effective if the whole of our lives, wakefulness and sleep, are not well balanced.
- Next, the timing of sleep has to be considered, and adjusted if necessary. This is a process of integrating our sleep patterns into the ebb and flow of our lives and the rhythms around us, especially the cycle of day and night and our biological rhythms.
- Having established the best timing for sleep, it's possible to improve the quality of the time spent asleep. This is done by eliminating the negative influences and disturbances, and naturally enhancing the nurturing elements.
- Finally, sleep is perfected by adjusting it to serve your best interests, to allow it to be as good as you dream that it could be.

We'll help you to achieve your fittest sleep by providing exactly what you need in ways that you can easily use. The cornerstone of this approach is the 'Twenty-one nights to better sleep' programme (see pages 56-164). This is an effective and tested programme that takes care of the details in a systematic way.

This book is in eight chapters, which, together, make up *The Sleep Solution*. In the first chapter, 'What is sleep?' we discuss sleep and its role in our lives. What happens when sleep goes wrong is covered in Chapter 2: 'Why you need better sleep'. We explain how to improve your sleep in a sensible way using the first three levels of improvement – damage control, the reactive level, and sleep fitness – in Chapter 3: 'Improving your sleep'. Then, in Chapter 4: 'Checking what's wrong with your sleep', there are questionnaires and guidelines so that you can discover how you are sleeping now and where you should focus your efforts for improvement. Chapter 5: 'Twenty-one nights to better sleep', is a tested, structured programme designed to bring about this sleep improvement. In Chapter 6: 'Creative sleep', we show how to use your sleep to enhance your life. A compendium of useful information about sleep and related problems is presented in Chapter 7: 'Sleep tips: help for specific sleep problems'. Finally, in Chapter 8: 'Sleep resources', we describe how to obtain further information.

You may be wondering how this book differs from the others next to it on the bookshelves. Choosing a book, like choosing a pillow, is obviously a very personal matter. But we do believe that *The Sleep Solution* has some useful ideas. We have tried hard to make it work for every individual who picks it up. This is a tall order: it is obviously easier to write in generalities which sound impressive but which omit the important details. Instead, we've tried to be comprehensive and we've checked the programme with people who have real sleep problems – people who suffer from complex problems as well as those with the minor irritations that don't interest most doctors.

We became interested in sleep because we found that it was fascinating. Nigel entered the field of sleep medicine after becoming aware of the large number of people who truly suffer from sleep disorders and rarely receive the treatment they deserve. We both moved into the positive health aspects of sleep when we realized that just treating the very sick is not the most effective answer. Our goal is to give people the opportunity to improve their sleep before they become really ill, lose their job, or even just end up in a different room from their partner at night. We hope that this is the sleep solution for you.

Nigel Ball, Seattle, Washington, USA
Nick Hough, London, UK
May 1999

CHAPTER 1

What is sleep?

S leep is compelling, mysterious, and wonderful. It is also misunderstood, much abused and, when poorly managed, can be dangerous. Before messing about with sleep, it's important to know something about it. Do you believe that you'll die if you don't get enough sleep, or that you don't have a sleep problem because you can sleep anywhere, at any time? Do you think that coffee doesn't affect your sleep, and that you're safe when you are sleepy at the wheel because you don't take chances? Do you know why you're sometimes groggy when you wake up but ready to go at other times? Understanding sleep will provide the right foundation for our programme to improve your sleep.

THE MERITS OF SLEEP

Many people, even some experts, have made the mistake of not being serious enough about their sleep. (Others may have been a little too serious.) Why do we sleep? Do we need to sleep? Let's examine the evidence.

Whichever way you look at it, sleep occupies an impressively large part of our lives. We sleep for almost a third of our time on this planet: on average, about 23 years. We spend more time asleep than we spend working, looking after children, exercising, talking, or even watching television. We spend more intimate time with ourselves in sleep than with all of our lovers or spouses, and there is a good chance that we will die in our sleep and be glad that it happens that way. Whatever else, sleep is a major feature of life on earth.

Why can't we do without sleep?

Why don't we spend the time that we now spend sleeping doing something more useful? Why can't we do without sleep? Some people have tried to beat the system and do this. Of course, it doesn't work if you go 'cold turkey' and suddenly stop sleeping. Most of us tried that once or twice when we were young and can still remember the horrible, growing sleepiness after one or two nights, and the relief to finally get to bed and go to sleep. The record is more than 260 hours without sleep, although most people can't manage a fraction of that time. But what if sleep were gradually eliminated, slowly squeezed from eight to four or even two hours? Many people have attempted this, but (as far as we know) no one has managed less than four hours on a regular basis because they find the side-effects of not getting enough sleep intolerable. (Incidentally, most people don't become psychotic after several days without sleep – that's a myth – but they don't feel very well either!)

Leonardo da Vinci tried a different approach to this problem. Rather than cutting down his main sleep period, he slept for twenty minutes every two hours, which adds up to about four hours in every day. Of course, as a philosopher and artist in fifteenth-century Renaissance Italy, his lifestyle allowed such an indulgence. You will note that even he didn't break the four-hour barrier, and it's also possible that his wakefulness may have been exaggerated over time.

In the Sleep Disorders Center in Seattle we ask the patients about the sleep patterns they would prefer in an ideal world. Of the last two thousand patients or so, two demanded lengthy sleep beginning 'right now', and the remainder proposed six to twelve hours starting between 8 p.m. and 2 a.m., and ending between 4 a.m. and noon. No one has asked for no sleep in his or her ideal world! None of these people could imagine a life in which they had an extra eight hours a day to do the things that they would love to do 'if only there were time'. None was willing to suggest swapping sleep for another career or an opportunity to move ahead of the competition.

Another sign that sleep is important comes from studying how sleep has evolved. Obviously, we can't dig up fossils to find out what sleep was like in the past. Instead, we try to draw conclusions from the sleep patterns of the variety of creatures that still live today. This is rather like astronomers examining the light from stars deep in other galaxies that died billions of years ago. Sleep, in one form or another, is a feature of all animals that have organs and nerves, from the simplest to the most elaborate. It's been at least 500 million years since animals first started to sleep, and yet there isn't a single species alive today that doesn't sleep. Apparently, sleep is too fundamental to be easily avoided, and too beneficial to have been given up.

Even people who sleep too much are proof that sleep is unavoidable. Many of them insist that they don't have a sleep problem because they could fall asleep at any time, wherever they are. Actually, the quality of their sleep is so poor that they have to be asleep for longer and longer just to try to compensate. They can't just eliminate the poor-quality sleep.

But what of people with insomnia? Surely these are people (and perhaps you're one) who are forced to get by with little or no sleep? To understand this, and to begin to grasp the essence of *The Sleep Solution,* we'll need to discuss the complexity and richness of sleep.

THE RICHNESS OF SLEEP

Sleep is not only essential, it's also well structured and well organized. It's not simply a deeper form of resting, just as sleepiness is not simply being extremely tired. It's complex, and this is something that we'll have to keep in mind as we strive to achieve perfect sleep.

What do we mean by 'sleep'? Many of us think of sleep as a period of nothingness somewhere between turning out the light and the alarm going off in the morning. If it works well we need little convincing that it's been refreshing and somewhat restorative. But what is happening while we are in the Land of Nod? Let's start by explaining what sleep is not.

What sleep is not

Sleep is *not* nothingness. It is not like putting the car in the garage, turning off the engine, closing the doors and leaving it until morning. When we are asleep, things *happen*, and these are different from the kinds of things that take place during the day. In sleep, our brains, cells and digestion can be as active as they were during the day, and our hearts can beat as fast. Sleep is not a 'mini death'. Nor is sleep the same as resting. Resting is a passive, gentle form of wakefulness. When we rest we are still awake. When we rest we are responsive and alert.

Sleep is not a sign of laziness, or an indication of weakness. We've all seen the 'I can drive all night and all day and not crash' mentality at work. Such people are playing Russian roulette with their lives and those of other people, and an accident is only a matter of time. The person who sleeps for twelve hours a night and still cannot stay awake at dinnertime is not simply lazy. Lazy people are usually far more content to do nothing than to sleep. No, these people have a sleep disorder that needs to be resolved.

What sleep is

We're asleep when we disconnect from our surroundings in a way that is easily and rapidly reversed, and that is controlled from within us. When we are asleep we're largely unconscious or unresponsive: we lose sensation, the ability to think properly, and our short-term memory. Clearly, it's not a complete separation from the outside world – a mother can still wake up when her child cries, for example – but it is a profound and swift change from the waking situation.

Sleep arises from within us, spontaneously, and is not just a response to things that happen to us. Somewhere in our brains or bodies exist systems to decide how much sleep we need, and when that sleep should occur. Sleep is not imposed on us like anaesthesia or hypnosis.

Sleep is rapidly reversible. It's possible, and usual, to be deeply asleep, yet within minutes to be fully awake. So sleep is different from hibernation or a coma.

Sometimes, especially when we are drowsy, it isn't clear if we're asleep or not. Sleep can intrude into wakefulness in tiny episodes lasting only a few seconds ('microsleeps'). A single microsleep can kill a sleepy driver (if you nod off at 70 m.p.h., you can travel almost 200 yards in five seconds) yet you may experience only a slight startle as you wake up again.

Typical sleep

A typical night's sleep isn't one continuous uniform period of sleep. It actually comprises four or five sleep cycles. Each cycle is an episode of sleep lasting between 90 and 120 minutes in which there is a gradual deepening of sleep and then a return to light sleep or, sometimes, brief wakefulness. The structure of these sleep cycles contributes to what sleep does, and to how it goes wrong.

Within each sleep cycle there are two main types of sleep, which are so well integrated that it wasn't until about 50 years ago that their differences began to be appreciated. The first type is generally known as non-REM sleep (NREMS), although it would be a lot simpler and easier if it were called by its other name, Quiet sleep.

Quiet sleep

Quiet sleep is, simply, the type of sleep in which the brain is at its most inactive. Not everything stops, however. The body is immobile and losing heat so there might be some sweating. Some glands are busy secreting hormones (the poorly named growth hormone, for example), and some digestion occurs. Some, but not all, cells are busy making proteins that may contribute to the repair of our bodies after a long day of activity.

The heart and circulation are under less stress in good Quiet sleep than when we're awake. Blood pressure, heart rate, and breathing rates are all at their lowest values so the heart works less hard. Urine production is down, so going to the lavatory more than once during the night is a sure indication of disturbed sleep. The brain isn't very active. There are large, slow brainwaves, which are a good sign that not much is going on. These are interspersed with two other types of electrical signals in the brain. One type (sleep spindles) indicate 'If anything important happens I will be able to respond', and another kind (K-complexes), 'I just received a signal which is certainly not important enough to wake me up'.

It would be a mistake to interpret this 'quietness' as a sign that nothing important is happening. Some people's Quiet sleep is polluted by evidence of wakeful activity. They have very unsatisfactory sleep and awaken unrefreshed and tired. The disruption takes the form of electrical waves, known as alpha waves, that wash over the usual brainwaves of Quiet sleep. Another indication of the importance of Quiet sleep is that it occurs quickly and prominently when someone ends a prolonged time without sleep.

Quiet sleep itself has a complex structure made up of various stages. Stage one usually marks the transition into sleep and, generally, a healthy person only spends a few minutes at a time in this stage. This is not high-quality sleep. Stage two is like a framework on which many of the important functions of sleep are to be found. It may blend almost imperceptibly with the other sleep stages, but can also occur in uninterrupted blocks of more than 30 minutes. In normal sleep, the deepest form of Quiet sleep follows stage two. This is Delta sleep, characterized by large, slow brainwaves. It is also known as stages three and four. Delta sleep appears to be sensitive to disturbance, being easily lost if sleep is disrupted. Children have the most Delta sleep – about a third of the time they spend asleep – and this proportion gets smaller as we age, dwindling to less than a tenth of our sleep by late middle age.

REM sleep

The second and most distinctive type of sleep is REMS (rapid eye-movement sleep), which occurs near the end of each of the four or five sleep cycles. Episodes of REMS last about 30 minutes, becoming longer and closer together towards the end of the night. REMS is a kind of 'brain sleep'. In REMS the brain is active, so active in fact that the body has to be mostly paralysed to prevent the damage that would occur if we acted out our dreams. This combination of an active brain in an immobile body so mystified the early sleep researchers that they called this state 'active sleep' or 'paradoxical sleep'.

There are several other interesting things that happen when we're in REMS. We lose our ability to control the temperature of our bodies and shivering and sweating cease. Our heartbeat and breathing become faster and more erratic. Because of the paralysis of the muscles that control our ribs we have to rely on our diaphragm to breathe, and this can be a serious problem for some obese people. Blood flows to the sexual organs of men and women, and men have erections. Doctors have used this phenomenon to study impotence: if he has an erection in REMS, the patient does not have a physical problem.

Sleep in the rest of the animal kingdom

Simple animals (worms and insects, for example) have simple sleep, a basic type of Quiet sleep, in which they are immobile and unresponsive, and their life-support systems are running at a reduced level. The least evolved creatures with backbones – fish and amphibians – have a slightly more complex form of Quiet sleep with some special brainwaves.

The biggest event in the evolution of sleep occurred some 300 million years ago. When the vertebrates finally conquered the land for full-time living, as opposed to the temporary excursions of the amphibians, the first mammals and the birds developed the ability to control their body temperature from within and also their sleep. Almost all living mammals, including the egg-laying mammals (the monotremes) have both Quiet sleep and REMS. Bats and opossums are the champion sleepers, with eighteen to nineteen hours of sleep a day; domestic cats are not far behind, sleeping for more than 12 hours a day. Among mammals, the shortest sleeper is said to be the giraffe, which sleeps for only two hours in every 24, but it is thought that they are drowsy nappers for much of the time. Birds sleep less and in much shorter episodes. Some birds sleep for only seconds or minutes at a time.

Not all animals sleep in the same way. Birds can sleep while flying or swimming, and sleep experts were astonished to learn that marine mammals (such as dolphins) and almost all birds can sleep with only one side of the brain at a time, while the other side remains awake. This is known as 'unihemispheric sleep'. This way of sleeping is clearly sensible for a mammal that breathes air but lives underwater: to be completely asleep and unable to swim to the surface for air would mean drowning! For birds, the advantage of unihemispheric sleep is that they can sleep and look out for predators simultaneously. Humans may have this ability to sleep with only part of the brain at a time, but certainly not to the same degree as dolphins and whales. Researchers are increasingly finding differences between parts of the brain during sleep, but not whole hemispheres at a time. Undoubtedly more research will be done in this area in the years to come.

How does the richness and complexity of sleep play a role in *The Sleep Solution?*

The richness of sleep is easy to see. It is ancient and robust. It is so much a part of our lives that we'll have to work with it, not against it to make the most of it and make it work for us. But how does this richness play a role in *The Sleep Solution?*

Perhaps the most significant implication is that we are poor judges of what is going on while we're asleep. We're unaware of our sleep cycles and sleep stages, and we can be equally unaware of snoring, pauses in our breathing, or even sleep-walking. To judge our sleep we have to rely on the observations of others, or, more importantly, draw conclusions from how we feel during the day.

Some sleep problems are linked to specific components of sleep. Through an understanding of the complexity of sleep you'll be able to appreciate, for example, the difference between sleep terrors and nightmares. You'll recognize that the grogginess you feel when awakening to answer the phone after you've been asleep for an hour is perfectly natural, and understand why breathing problems are often worse later in the night.

THE CONTROL OF SLEEP

Funnily enough, to understand how well sleep controls wakefulness, we have to start with how sleep itself is controlled. A key concept of *The Sleep Solution* is that sleep controls wakefulness, and wakefulness controls sleep. There are two main ways in which wakefulness controls sleep: the delicate balance between how much sleep we need and how much sleep we've achieved (the sleep-wake balance), and the daily biological rhythm that we call the circadian rhythm.

The sleep-wake balance
The longer we've been awake, the more we need to sleep and the more likely we are to fall asleep. This makes good sense. Similarly, if we miss some sleep one night (getting up early, for example), we need more sleep on the next night. Sleep seems to respond to a need that comes from our waking activities.

You've probably noticed that you don't need exactly the same number of hours of sleep to catch up as you lost originally. This is because sleep is almost always more intense for the first few hours than later in the sleep period. So during the recovery night we sleep more deeply and need less time to catch up.

Circadian rhythms
If we just slept whenever we accumulated a sleep debt, we would be forever falling asleep. Our sleep patterns would resemble those of a newborn baby: sleep, eat, smile, sleep, eat, smile, etc. As adults it makes more sense to time things so that we sleep at night when our waking

activities are limited, work in the morning when our minds and bodies are fresh, and relax in the evening. How do we accommodate this kind of patterning and impose some structure on the other physiological activities that need to be correctly timed? Each of us has a basic biological rhythm of body temperature, highest after midday and lowest at 3 to 5 a.m. This does not depend on what we do, but is reset each day by the sun's light. Under normal circumstances, our sleep is synchronized to this pattern and we find it easier to fall asleep when our body temperature is falling in the late evening and easiest to wake up when we're warming up in the morning. This is why most people like to fall asleep between 10 p.m. and midnight and why night-workers who go to bed at 8 a.m. often wake up, to their frustration, between 11 a.m. and 1 p.m. The early afternoon is a second opportunity for sleep. At this time the body temperature is high enough for us to throttle back on metabolic rate. This allows us to go to sleep.

People who have a naturally early circadian rhythm are known as 'larks'. These people like to get up early, and do their best work in the morning. At the other extreme are the 'night owls', who like to stay up late, and feel at their best during the evening. Too much has been made of the distinction between these types, however. Most people have some preference about bedtime but may not have a corresponding 'best time of day'. It's wise to be aware of this relationship, but on the whole it doesn't work to force individuals into such rigid categories.

The forbidden zone

There is a time, perhaps two to three hours before normal bedtime, when it's extremely difficult to fall asleep. This has been termed 'the forbidden zone'. Of course, people with sleep problems or disorders, and especially those who are habitually sleep-deprived, can sleep at this time, or doze in front of the television, but most of us find it difficult. This is one of the reasons why it is harder to go to bed earlier than the usual time. Many people notice this most strongly when, after going to bed late on Friday and Saturday night, they try to get an early night on Sunday and have difficulty falling asleep.

Debt and rhythm

These two influences, the sleep-wake balance and the circadian rhythm, combine to control the patterns of wakefulness and sleep. Let's consider the typical pattern of someone – Jane for example – who is awake during the day and sleeping at night. Jane wakes in the morning on her rising temperature rhythm, having restored her sleep-wake balance by seven hours of deep, restful sleep. Since she is awake and active she's beginning to accumulate a need for sleep, but as her temperature continues to rise through the day she is able to remain alert and sharp. Just after lunch some of this growing need for sleep breaks through because her digestion makes her more sluggish, but overall she does well until she starts to unwind in the evening. Her temperature is now falling, and she's ready for sleep. She gets into bed and sleeps soundly for another seven hours. And so it continues.

Why do teenagers want to go to bed late and get up late, while many older people feel ready for bed in the mid-evening? This is mainly because circadian rhythms tend to be delayed (that is, late) when we are young, and advanced (early) as we age. Some people also have an unnaturally late circadian rhythm, which means that they never feel ready for sleep before 2 or 3 a.m., and are never ready to get up before 10 or 11 a.m. This disorder is known as 'Delayed sleep phase syndrome'. The lucky ones find careers in which they can work during the evening or at night. The forbidden zone makes it difficult for the others to get to sleep on time and they have substantial problems getting to work on time. Some use bright-light therapy, others try to delay their sleep by an hour a day until an appropriate bedtime is achieved.

Five-day patterns
On a daily basis we have some capacity to adjust for various degrees of sleep need. So if we're late one night because of a social engagement, we may still be able to keep a reasonably normal schedule the next day. But, sooner or later, the debt will need to be repaid. Some calculations that we've done in Seattle indicate that a five- to seven-day average of sleep is the most informative. In other words, five days is about as long as a mild sleep debt can be incurred without either daytime sleepiness or recovery (catch-up) sleep becoming necessary.

Weekends

The five-day pattern may well explain the origin of the week and the concept of the weekend. If it's not possible for human beings to go longer than five days without catch-up sleep, early peoples moving from an open schedule to an era of responsibility may have settled naturally for a scheme which provided a built-in day or two of rest.

SLEEP, THE GREAT CONTROLLER

Sleep also controls wakefulness. In fact, sleep is the Great Controller, magnifying and changing what we do when we are awake. This is something you'll need to think about and use in improving your sleep.

Sleep begins its work for the next day almost as soon as we fall asleep. By disconnecting our minds from the outside – that uninterrupted flow of sensory stimulation – the brain can restabilize some systems. Stressful activation can be calmed. Those messages which are sent to release the hormones that keep us on edge can be slowly reduced. Brain circuits that have been heavily used receive a welcome respite. The brain and body move into a secure mode that requires little by way of constant adjustment or responding to the environment.

Once this process is well under way, more active work can begin. Hormones can be released to fine-tune the body and take care of some processes that would otherwise interfere with what we're doing when we're awake. Memories can be consolidated and some learning can be finalized. It's possible that the brain takes stock of what's been happening and adjusts itself so that it's ready to perform better during the forthcoming day. This may be what goes on during REMS.

Finally, preparation for waking up and getting the day going can begin. Just as it's essential for us to wind down at night in order to sleep properly, it's also essential to gear up correctly for the day ahead. Some hours before we wake up, physiological changes are already taking place. Activating hormones are released, our heart rate begins to rise, and our circuits start to get ready. There may be a short period of grogginess on first awakening, but with good sleep the brain and body are ready for the day ahead within minutes.

WHAT DOES ALL THIS MEAN FOR *THE SLEEP SOLUTION?*

> **How you will feel and behave tomorrow depends on how you sleep tonight.**

This one sentence summarizes what we think sleep is about, and conveys the overall message of this book. If you change the way you think about your sleep, then perhaps for the first time, you will understand that you can control your sleep and improve your life.

The huge changes and advances of the twentieth century have left us with lives that would be barely recognizable to someone living a hundred years ago: electric lights, clock radios, computers, televisions, VCRs, rapid intercontinental travel, and sophisticated healthcare. But what have we done for our sleep? Ignored it! Now many of us are paying the price for our neglect, and are finding that our lives and health are suffering.

In this chapter we've outlined what sleep is. Now we'll describe what happens when sleep goes wrong and what you should do to put it right.

CHAPTER 2

Why you need better sleep

S leep can appear to be a mixture of the fragile and the heavy-handed. Some people are victims of the fragility of sleep when the slightest upsetting incident during the day triggers a sleepless, clock-watching night. Others are more aware of its demanding interference. No matter how much time they spend asleep, they always feel groggy and unrested during the day. To fully appreciate the benefits you can expect from fitter sleep, you should first understand what happens when there are problems with sleep.

WHEN SLEEP GOES WRONG

When sleep goes wrong, bad things happen. Over the last fifteen years it's become clear that many of us are not sleep-healthy. A recent Gallup poll in the United States showed that about a third of the population have problems with their sleep. Only about one in five of us have good, untainted sleep.

Sleep disorders

Who has never had **insomnia**? For some it's a difficulty with falling asleep, for others staying asleep, or getting back to sleep. It is the most common sleep problem and it affects about a third of us each year in some form or another. About one in seven people have insomnia that is severe enough to affect their lives or health, and one in eleven have insomnia almost every night for six months at a time.

It's difficult to generalize about insomnia because it's a symptom and so has many possible causes. Pain, discomfort, stress, an excitable nature, depression, hormone imbalance, anxiety, poor sleep habits, and unhealthy living can all contribute to insomnia. It is a feature of many different disorders.

For most insomnia problems there are predisposing, precipitating and perpetuating factors. A predisposing factor might be an anxious personality, either naturally or perhaps as a result of psychological trauma when young. A precipitating factor might have been an illness or stressful period. The perpetuating factor might be the noise in a bedroom that is too close to a motorway.

Significantly, people with insomnia often adopt habits that make their problem worse. Perhaps that's why it's such a difficult problem to cure. Basically, we have to 'let go' at some level in order to get to sleep. Once you've experienced difficulty getting to sleep, you'll be slightly less confident that you'll get to sleep the next time, and so on. This applies to possible cures too, so that the insomnia sufferer will often try, and persist with, treatments that just don't seem to overcome the problems of getting to sleep.

Insomnia is more likely to be experienced by some people than others. Women have insomnia more often than men, and poor people are more likely to have insomnia than rich people. Insomnia is a particular problem for those who have been abused, or suffered severe trauma. For some people it's a harmless but frustrating problem, for others it leads to poor health and a miserable life.

The second most common sleep disorder is **insufficient sleep syndrome**. Not only is this a sleep disorder, but many experts believe that almost all of us would do better with more sleep. Obviously, we think here of mothers with small children and busy professionals, but most schoolchildren, young professionals and elderly people also need more sleep. The solution is not quite as simple as spending more time in bed, although that would help millions of people. A better approach is covered in some detail in the 'Twenty-one nights to better sleep' programme (see pages 56-164).

About 10 per cent of men and five per cent of women have significant **breathing problems** while they sleep. These breathing problems range from harmless light snoring to complete pauses, which are known as apnoeas. These pauses can last from a few seconds to a couple of minutes and, at worst, occur hundreds of times each hour. With each pause there is a partial or complete obstruction to breathing, leading to a drop in the oxygen content of the blood and hence less oxygen going to the brain. The body reacts quickly and slows the heart and drops the blood pressure. As the obstruction is breached (often with a snort or a gasp from the sleeper), there is a short arousal and the heart races and the blood pressure rises in an attempt to restore the oxygen supplies quickly. Over time this **obstructive sleep apnoea** leads to extensive sleepiness while awake, and such health problems as high blood pressure, heart attacks, or even stroke. The brain may be irreparably damaged: it's just not possible for it to recover from years of depleted oxygen for several hours a day. Recently, experts have been wondering whether the partial obstructions to breathing that occur with intermittent 'crescendo' snoring are also somewhat harmful. This has been called the **upper airway resistance syndrome**.

Why is it difficult to breathe when we're asleep? There's no single reason. As we breathe in, we always reduce the pressure in our lungs to suck in air from the outside. When we're asleep, we're more relaxed, so this pressure also tends to pull in or vibrate the airway, causing snoring. If there are other influences that make the airway smaller or less rigid, the airway can be pulled in enough to impede or even stop the flow of air, as in apnoea (which, incidentally, is Greek for 'want of breath').

The airway may be naturally narrow, or made smaller by extra body weight, nasal congestion, a large uvula (the dangly bit at the back of your mouth), prominent tonsils, or a receding jaw. The things that make the airway less rigid include increasing age, tiredness and alcohol consumption. It's been said that over three-quarters of the breathing problems in sleep that we're so concerned about today are caused by obesity.

There are two other things that make snoring and apnoea worse. One is sleeping on your back, which makes breathing more difficult because your gut presses against your diaphragm. The second is REMS. You'll recall that in REM sleep many of our muscles are paralysed. This includes the rib muscles and some of the muscles around the airway, which means that not only are you breathing only with your diaphragm in REMS, but also the airway is floppier and easy to collapse.

There are several sleep disorders that are each found in two to six per cent of the population. **Periodic limb movement disorder** is usually noticed only by the sleeper's partner, because the sleeper is asleep and unaware of it. In this disorder, repetitive twitching or kicking movements of the limbs (usually the legs) occur every 10 to 40 seconds or so during periods of the night. While not dangerous in themselves, they disrupt sleep and cause unwelcome sleepiness, both for the mover and often for the partner! Again, there is no single cause, but this problem is intensified by caffeine, sleep deprivation, anaemia, and kidney problems.

Restless legs syndrome is a disorder that the sufferers describe in a myriad ways, but which is obvious to anyone who has experienced it. It is the restless, itchy, burning feeling of the legs which is relieved only by movement and which tends to occur when the sufferer is tired and nearly ready to go to sleep. One patient described it as though 'my skin has been taken off,' and sand glued to my bare flesh, and then the skin put back on'. Other people talk in terms of insects, or burning. The severity of the sensation may prevent the sufferer from getting to sleep, and it may even provoke mental problems and lead to suicide. Sufferers are generally unaware that there are several medicines for this problem, and most cases have not been correctly diagnosed or treated. The disorder is more severe in people who have kidney conditions or blood problems, such as anaemia, who suffer from sleep deprivation, or have a high caffeine consumption. It is much worse with sleep deprivation or exhaustion. People with restless legs syndrome often also have periodic limb movement disorder, but are usually unaware of it.

In addition to these common disorders, there are some rarer problems that are worth mentioning because of their impact on the lives of those afflicted, and those of their partners and family members. **Narcolepsy** is a relatively rare disorder, experienced by fewer than six in every thousand people. It is dramatic and devastating for the afflicted until they are diagnosed and the treatment begins. The usual pattern is one of more than ten years between the onset of the disease and the start of appropriate treatment, often ten years of fear and suffering. People with narcolepsy are extremely sleepy during the day, usually with irresistible sleep attacks. These are the classic 'fall asleep while eating' people, although some people with severe sleep apnoea can be equally sleepy.

Many sufferers of narcolepsy have three other symptoms that are frightening and bizarre. First, they sometimes see hallucinations at bedtime. These can be visions of people in the room (ghosts, or evil strangers bending over the bed), or animals such as dogs or rabbits. Children tend to see colourful animals. Second, on awakening they may find that they're completely paralysed for up to a few minutes, or perhaps able to move only their eyes. They usually become very afraid, fearing that they might have had a stroke, or perhaps that they'll never wake up. Finally, and often later in the development of the disease, they may experience a sudden weakness when emotional, laughing or angry. This can be so extreme that the person collapses to the floor in a paralysed state, and needs to sleep. One patient had this experience whenever a stranger in a grocery store talked to her. She became almost a recluse as a result, until we arranged the correct treatment. (It should be emphasized that people without narcolepsy can have any of these symptoms in isolation, so an occasional episode of sleep paralysis does not mean that you have or will develop narcolepsy.)

People with narcolepsy might have been incorrectly told that they are suffering from seizures, depression or schizophrenia, or that they're just plain lazy, so a prompt visit to a sleep disorders specialist is certainly called for.

There are many different disorders involving unwanted activity in sleep, but we've only space to address three of them. The first involves a sudden burst from bed, perhaps with screaming or yelling and a dash to the door. The sleeper may remember nothing about this, or may be aware of terror, a racing heart, and a sense of doom or fear. This can be a **night terror** or a **panic attack**. Both are exacerbated by stress, sleep apnoea, disrupted sleep, and too much caffeine. Both can be treated.

The second is **nocturnal eating disorder**. We mention this because we suspect that it's a lot more common than is usually reported, and results in much anguish for the sufferers. Basically, the person gets up during the night, either when fully asleep or partly asleep, and eats. This may be moderately sensible eating, such as sweets or biscuits, or it may be more bizarre: eating paper towels smeared with peanut butter, for example. Sometimes the patient is aware of the disorder only because of the food debris they find in the bed in the morning; it may be covered in chocolate or jam, perhaps. Sometimes this is dangerous. Patients have cut themselves preparing food with sharp knives, and they commonly burn things in the microwave or on the cooker.

Finally, there is the disorder of acting out dreams while asleep. This sounds funny, but it can be the most sinister of sleep disorders. Unfortunately, the dreams are often violent, and occasionally partners have been killed after getting involved in a situation in which the sleeper, ironically, was dreaming that he was protecting his partner from attack by someone else. This disorder is called **REM sleep behaviour disorder**, reflecting the sleep stage in which it occurs. It responds fairly well to treatment with medication.

There are many other sleep disorders. All affect health and well-being to some degree, but it's not necessary to have a formal sleep disorder to have unsatisfactory sleep. Even minor sleep problems can affect your health.

THE IMPACT OF SLEEP ON HEALTH

Broadly speaking, sleep problems affect health and well-being in one of two ways. Sleep problems can cause sleepiness, either directly or as a result of disrupted sleep, and this sleepiness can then lead to accidents and poor performance. Second, disrupted sleep can damage some basic life processes, such as the circulation and digestion.

Sleepiness

Many sleep problems cause sleepiness, and sleepiness contributes to bad health through accidents and injury. Sleepiness is the intrusion of sleep-like processes into waking activity.

Not all sleepiness is bad: imagine trying to fall asleep if you could never experience the sensation of sleepiness. That kind of sleepiness is called **useful sleepiness**. When we talk about the sleepiness that comes from sleep problems, we're usually referring to a kind of **unwelcome sleepiness**, a sleepiness that gets in the way of what we'd like to do.

Often, things that you might think cause sleepiness (such as a warm room, boredom, or monotony) are actually only allowing the sleepiness that was already present to become obvious. Similarly, it's hard to get rid of sleepiness without going to sleep, although it may be less evident if you're active or interested in something.

Unwelcome sleepiness should not be confused with lethargy, the 'don't want to do anything' of stress, depression, and boredom, even though lethargy is often accompanied by sleepiness. Nor should it be confused with fatigue, which is the 'can't do anything' feeling we get with medical problems such as infectious illnesses. Generally, sleepy people want to sleep, or feel better if they do sleep. However, many people with sleep disorders (especially insomnia) also feel fatigued. Governments and transportation industries are increasingly using fatigue as an all-encompassing term. Chronic fatigue syndrome is a specific (and rather over-diagnosed) disorder of fatigue that has persisted for at least six months with significant disability and with no evidence of a sleep disorder.

Sleepiness is not simple. Some people say that they don't feel sleepy but clearly *are* sleepy because they can't stay awake to watch a film, they listen to music to keep themselves alert when they're driving, drink pots of coffee, stand up to read, or make mistakes at work. There's more about these types of sleepiness later in the book, but for now note that you don't have to feel sleepy to be sleepy.

Sleepiness causes accidents. It's reckoned that 30 to 50 per cent of all accidents are the result of sleepiness, and that sleepiness is a particular factor in fatal accidents. You're probably very aware of the major accidents or near accidents such as the Chernobyl and *Exxon Valdez* disasters, which can be attributed to sleep-related incidents. However, huge as those were, the constant everyday toll in lives and property is greater. The numbing tragedy of the Hagley School minibus crash on the M6 in November 1993 in which twelve schoolchildren and their teacher were killed as a result of the driver apparently falling asleep at the wheel is echoed many times every day in less dramatic fashion.

Sleepiness reduces productivity. Where companies have been able to improve wakefulness, even a little, productivity has risen by over 20 per cent. Again, more poignant influences may be apparent at the individual rather than the corporate level. Sleepiness results in poorer social skills, negative moods, a greater likelihood of divorce, fewer promotions, and ultimately, less success in life.

How sleep disruption affects health

Sleep disorders kill. Several studies have shown that, over a five- or ten-year period, people who have poor sleep are more likely to die than those who have good sleep. Furthermore, the best predictor of death in one group studied was the number of hours of sleep each obtained: both too few and too many hours of sleep proved to be unhealthy.

One reason for this mortality rate is that disrupted sleep intensifies problems with the heart and circulation. Up to three times the rate of strokes and five times the rate of heart attacks occur in people with poor sleep. This is not just among the old or disabled; younger people are similarly afflicted.

Why does sleep, or lack of sleep, affect the heart and circulation in this way? First, many people have poor sleep because of breathing problems such as snoring or sleep apnoea. As we've discussed, these problems increase blood pressure and damage the heart. Second, sleep disruption is stressful, and stress reactions take their toll. So, even those who just sleep poorly (without breathing problems) may have higher cholesterol and blood pressure levels than would otherwise be expected. Finally, when our sleep is disrupted, we lose our restful, restorative eight hours of sleep a day. This is almost like growing older at up to one and a half times the normal rate – probably as good a reason as any for sorting out your sleep before it's too late.

There are other health issues which might not be as lethal as the problems of the heart and circulation, but which are costly and upset the quality of life. The digestive system is particularly vulnerable. Stress and lack of rest also affect this. But the digestive system is strongly controlled by biological rhythms and activity patterns, and not just by what, and when, we eat. This means that when those patterns of sleep and activity are disrupted – as happens with most sleep problems – the digestive system may find itself with plenty of corrosive acids and enzymes but no food. These will start to work on the lining of the stomach and intestines. Later on, there may be food but no means to deal with it, which is another unhealthy situation. These problems are particularly severe for people who travel across time zones or have variable or disrupted schedules, for example, those with young children who eat at all hours.

Breathing problems also play havoc with the digestive system. The fluctuations in breathing of apnoea and upper airway resistance syndrome cause pressure changes in the chest which then suck acids out of the stomach and into the oesophagus or, worse still, into the lungs. This burning acid disrupts sleep (even if the sleeper is unaware of it), causes coughing, and damages the lining of the oesophagus.

One of the first casualties from poor sleep is mood. Almost universally, poor sleepers become more irritable. Many people with sleep problems are also depressed. In a sleep disorders centre it's common to hear the patients say, 'I don't have depression, I'm just depressed because I'm tired'.

People who suffer from insomnia are often anxious. We tend to assume that the anxiety causes the insomnia, but a case could also be made that poor sleep contributes to their anxiety. Certainly, a cure for disrupted sleep can take the edge off an anxious personality.

Surprisingly, shortened sleep (but not disrupted sleep) can improve the mood of some people who have depression. Most of us have occasionally experienced an elevated mood from deep sleep and an early awakening.

What this means for you

Regardless of whether or not your health or well-being have already been seriously compromised by poor sleep, you probably have some concerns about your sleep and know that most sleep problems get worse with time. How should you set about improving your sleep? We'll tell you how in the next chapter.

CHAPTER 3

Improving your sleep

As you've probably already discovered, it's rarely helpful to tackle your sleep problems in a half-hearted fashion. Cures or treatments that ought to work don't, or they work for a while and then, mysteriously, become ineffective. Your 'medicine cabinet' is full of part-used pill bottles, as it were.

If you're going to improve your sleep you'll need to be organized and systematic. Urgent problems must be dealt with quickly and the longer-term issues more comprehensively. There are four main levels.

The first level is for **damage control**. Here you'll take immediate care of pressing problems such as dangerous sleepiness. At the **reactive level** you will be finding solutions to those sleep disorders which materially affect either your life or your health. You'll need to react to these problems to get back to normal. The third level is for **sleep fitness**. At this level you may feel generally healthy and do reasonably well. However, you're aware of certain sleep problems that are inconvenient or troublesome. A cure might have been worse than the disease. Or perhaps your sleep has been limited, so that you are OK only if you go to bed early. By taking care of these problems you'll achieve more satisfaction from your sleep. Finally, at the **creative level** there is an understanding that life can be, and should be, exploited for greater benefit. The emphasis is on flexibility, adaptability, and performance. This might be as simple as getting a few extra things done each week, or as rewarding as finally expressing your artistic or creative nature, even while you're still coping with a busy life.

There are also some things that you will do at each of these levels.

These are **rebalancing**, **timing**, **quality**, and **perfecting**. Let's examine each of these in a little more detail.

As sleep is an integral part of your whole life, no sleep solution will be effective if the time you spend awake is not also taken into account. For most people this means **rebalancing** their wakeful activities. This is a practical issue that surfaces all the time in the treatment of sleep disorders, and one that makes a tremendous difference if taken seriously. The concept is quite simple: the things that happen when you're awake affect sleep. If you neglect your waking time, your sleep will suffer. The easiest way to sort out your waking time is to ensure that you have the right balance of the main types of activities.

Let's take an example. A patient has great difficulty getting to sleep because her mind is too active. She worries about her finances and her work. When asked about the balance of her life it is clear that she does almost nothing except work and worry about her family. If she added some other interests, she would have more pleasant things to think about and to anticipate, and she would be more likely to meet people who would provide a sense of perspective about her troubles, and who might even support her.

The **timing** of sleep has to be corrected. Some people don't allow themselves enough opportunity to get the sleep they need because they're just not in bed for long enough. Others are in bed for too long so that their sleep is stretched and of poor quality. A third group are in bed for long enough, but the timing of their sleep is poor. They might be going to bed during the 'forbidden zone' when it's very difficult to get to sleep, or else in the morning after working all night when waking will be almost inevitable within a few hours. Inadequate sleep will almost certainly result from these kinds of timing mistakes.

Many sleep problems become worse over time leading to bad sleep habits, and creating other types of poor sleep. The first step in any successful sleep programme is to prevent this vicious cycle. Establishing the correct opportunity for sleep, both in terms of *when* and *for how long* is essential.

It's not always easy to sleep when we'd like to. How does the young mother pattern her sleep if she has a newborn baby who is awake for most of the night, and a two-year-old demanding her attention during the day? Or a working parent whose spouse keeps irregular hours? How to get the right timing and patterning for your sleep in a variety of circumstances is explained in the 'Twenty-one nights to better sleep' programme (see pages 56–164).

Once the correct timing of sleep has been established, you should work on the **quality** of the time you spend asleep. This involves eliminating disturbances and bad influences and nurturing the positive elements. At the reactive level, for example, this means finding the right treatment or natural therapy for the sleep disorders from which you suffer. At the sleep-fitness level it means taking care of those everyday issues that interfere with your sleep.

A case history will illustrate this. A patient was having a hard time getting to sleep and staying asleep during the night. She had developed a form of insomnia in which bad habits (such as going to bed too early) perpetuated her difficulty in getting to sleep. She also slept with three cats on her bed. Both of these issues needed to be resolved before she was able to sleep well again.

Finally, your sleep is **perfected** by adjusting it to create better wakeful living. You'll begin to perfect your sleep when you do the right things to ensure decent sleep in the future, whether you have a sleep problem or not. This is similar to the concept of fitness conditioning in sports.

A PRACTICAL APPROACH TO IMPROVING YOUR SLEEP

One successful approach is to address each level (damage control, reactive, sleep fitness, and creative) in turn, and that's the approach we'll use. We'll cover the first three levels in this chapter, and leave the creative level for Chapter 6.

DAMAGE CONTROL

> **'I need help and I need it now.'**

Many people have sleep problems so extreme that an extended programme, even if it does get to the root of the problem, is quite unacceptable. These problems may not be the most severe, just the most urgent. Perhaps you've been worn down by your insomnia, for example, and last night was the final straw. Perhaps coping is becoming increasingly difficult. As we discussed earlier, coping skills are some of the first victims of poor sleep.

The details differ, but there are some things that you'll need to think about whatever the problem is. These are:

- safety
- sleep
- other people
- starting over

Let's look at a few examples.

'I'm driving but I'm too sleepy to be safe. My head has nodded once or twice, and I've drifted across the road. It's only another fifteen miles until I get home.'

The chances are that you're already having microsleeps, which are extremely dangerous. At this degree of sleepiness you may be managing to drive, unless something unexpected happens (a child runs into the road, or the car in front stops suddenly). But as you become sleepier .... You've probably already started to do some things to make yourself more alert, such as opening the windows or turning up the radio. We've known people who have done exercises, pinched themselves, rolled a toy along the dashboard, or driven with their head out of the window. They've held a large container of icy water in their lap, or even got the passenger to steer while they operated the foot pedals. Scientific experiments have shown that measures such as these are clearly ineffective at reducing sleepiness to safe levels. Sadly, we've also known people who have had minor accidents, written-off cars, or ploughed into and killed pedestrians.

These self-rousing activities are not, usually, enough. So the first thing to do is to *stop*, in this case, literally. Obviously, you have to find a safe place. Remember that you'll almost always underestimate your sleepiness, and that some people have fallen completely asleep without any warning whatsoever. You should be thinking in terms of minutes, not tens of minutes. It's better to anticipate this need: it's awful to be trying to decide between a dangerous stopping place and more dangerous driving.

The hardest part of this process is convincing yourself that you're too sleepy. It's too easy to tell yourself, 'Just a few more miles' or, 'I've been like this before and I didn't crash'. But the sleepier you are, the more your judgement is impaired. How many last thoughts have been these, or 'I can make it'?

Once you've stopped, try to sleep. The most effective way of combating unwelcome sleepiness is to have a nap. Try napping in the car for ten or twenty minutes and leave yourself enough time to wake up fully when you're ready to start driving again. Can you involve other people? In this case, the easiest thing is to get someone else to drive, someone who's less sleepy than you are. If that's not possible, consider stopping for the night.

Perhaps you can't sleep safely where you are. The next best approach is to take a break, and drink some coffee. Caffeine takes a few minutes to start working, so it's a good idea to shake off some of your sleepiness in the meantime by getting some fresh air, moving around and getting a change of scene. You might also use this time to make your driving easier, by cleaning your windscreen, for example.

Finally, you should review your situation. Avoid the drowsy thinking that was obviously present before. Maybe you can rearrange your travel plans in order to stop sooner. Schedule your next break so that you have a decent meal and some time away from staring at the headlights or the white lines.

Remember, sleepiness kills, and the inconvenience of an early night at a motel is nothing compared to the inconvenience of a suspended driver's licence or much worse.

'I haven't slept in days. I'm desperate for some sleep. I just can't go on.'
Perhaps it's because of your children, or perhaps your mind won't switch off. Whatever the reason, you've been getting only a few hours' sleep each night and you're at the end of your tether. You need some immediate help to get you through this day or this night.

Stop anything you're doing that needs your full attention. If you're working, decide whether it's possible for you to go home. Perhaps you could take some time off sick. If you're looking after children, can you get some help, or at least meet up with a friend and spend some time together?

Next, decide whether you would be able to sleep right away. If you're sure that you won't be able to go to sleep, at least give yourself 20 or 30 minutes of relaxation and rest. You'll know what form it should take. Some people like to watch television, others to read, listen to music, or lie down in a sunny spot. Don't expect too much from this time: you're not going to solve all your problems in 30 minutes but, with luck, you should be slightly clearer-headed and more relaxed.

At the end of that time you'll need to begin to sort out a plan. This is often easier if you involve others, perhaps a good friend. You should recognize that you're almost certainly getting more sleep than you think you are at night, and that the road to recovery will be 'a day at a time'. Your plan should focus on specific issues, such as, 'How will I make dinner?' not, 'How can I go on?' You should make some decisions about resolving this problem for good. Will you carry out the programme outlined in this book, consult your doctor, or see a sleep specialist?

'I wish I could wake up fast in the morning.'
Many people are groggy when they wake up. It's all right if the feeling persists until you've had a shower, or even until your first cup of tea. But what should you do if you are still groggy when you are driving or at work? The ultimate solution to this problem lies with your night's sleep, but that doesn't help if you're already groggy. So what are the emergency measures to adopt?

If the grogginess is severe, or you have the opportunity (on the bus, for example), you can sneak a short nap. If you're dangerously sleepy, don't drive until you feel more alert. If you can't nap or you're still feeling groggy, take control of your schedule. Reschedule any critical tasks. Organize your time into short blocks, including as much variation and physical activity as you can. Do as many routine, unimportant jobs as possible.

If you have to attend a meeting or seminar, for instance, remember to use caffeine judiciously. Seek out light. If the room is dark, head for the outdoors (or at least to a window) for your breaks. Sip iced water during the session. If you still can't manage to be alert, you may be able to stand rather than sit. Focus on why you are there, and save your concentration for the most important issues.

'I have difficulty slowing down in the evening.'

The secret of slowing down in the evening is to establish a good routine. Get your brain used to a well-structured time that progresses from the stressful and the active through to the relaxing and the calming. Such a schedule works best if you anticipate future needs and deal with them early. For example, there may be some things that you may need to accomplish before the next day, such as paying bills or preparing clothes to wear. Do these early on and get them out of the way. This particularly applies to telephone calls. Try to finish using the telephone an hour or two before bedtime.

It's best if things that will affect your physiology, such as eating or exercise, are as routinely scheduled as possible. It's hard for your brain to adjust to a stressful day if it also has to deal with the effects of an early meal one day and a late one the next.

Don't assume that your current routine is the best or the most innocuous. Perhaps the coffee or wine that you drink with dinner does interfere with your sleep. You may be more affected by watching television than you think. These issues are dealt with in more detail later.

Try to arrange something pleasant to look forward to late in the evening. This can be reading, listening to music, or a quiet time in front of the fire.

THE REACTIVE LEVEL

> **'I have a little problem … .'**

At this level we're dealing with specific sleep disorders and problems. These are the kinds of issues that you know are affecting your health and well-being. For many, as we've discussed before, you should see your doctor or a sleep disorders specialist. Many others are so specific that you will need to use the materials in Chapter 7: 'Sleep tips: help for specific sleep problems'. You'll also benefit from the 'Twenty-one nights to better sleep' programme in Chapter 5; indeed, it might be a crucial part of your recovery. Often, sleep disorders are also associated with poor sleep habits and other problems with sleep. It can be difficult to resolve a sleep disorder without taking care of those issues.

Insomnia

The 'Twenty-one nights to better sleep' programme is ideally suited to help you to deal with many kinds of insomnia. It covers the basics to provide a firm foundation on which to make improvements, and also tackles the more specific issues that can upset a less comprehensive approach.

Before you begin such a programme, make sure that your general health is good, or, at least, is receiving the treatment that it deserves. If you haven't had a check-up for a while (generally once every three years for the under-40s, once every two years for the 40- to 50-year-olds, and annually thereafter), make an appointment. But don't delay starting the programme because you feel unwell, overweight, or 'in transition'.

There are some types of insomnia that won't be resolved completely using this programme, especially insomnia that has resulted from psychological trauma. Your sleep will improve, but to be cured you'll also need to treat the hurt that came from that emotional, physical or sexual abuse, or other psychologically traumatic event. Counselling or therapy can be extremely helpful, if not essential. Similarly, if you're in a bad relationship now, seek help.

Finally, you may be the naturally light sleeper or 'short-sleeper' who does not seem to need much sleep to do well when awake. You might have a driven, or what is called 'hyperarousable', personality. Again, don't judge your sleep need from some artificial standard or by comparing yourself with others. If you're clearly doing well in the daytime, and extending your sleep for a few days doesn't seem to make much difference, don't worry if you sleep less than other people.

Snoring and sleep apnoea

It's important to recognize that the intensity of treatment these problems require will depend on how severe they are.

At the simplest level, you may be a terrible snorer but have no unwelcome sleepiness, and no indication that your health is suffering. You don't have high blood pressure and you've never suffered from heart problems. This is primarily a social problem (people have been shot or divorced for snoring) and we make several suggestions about how to cope in Chapter 7.

Most people with notable sleep apnoea will have unwelcome sleepiness and perhaps some heart or circulation problems. At the personal level, the 'Twenty-one nights to better sleep' programme will be important in improving your overall sleep. You should also consider improving your general health, and, especially, taking sensible measures to reduce or control your weight. Your doctor will make sure that there's no immediately treatable problem such as a thyroid deficiency, but if your apnoea is severe enough he or she will recommend nasal CPAP (continuous positive airway pressure). This keeps the nose and throat open by blowing room air at a slight positive pressure through a mask into the nose and so into the airway. The latest developments are such devices which adjust their pressure during the night according to need.

There are few alternatives to CPAP. Apnoea is an unusual disorder in that surgery, in this case laser or conventional surgery of the uvula and palate, is suitable for the milder cases, not the most severe. For those with the right configuration of the jaw and throat – generally those with large tongues and small or receding jaws – orthodontic devices that fit around the teeth and hold the jaw and tongue forward are helpful.

Restless legs syndrome

Once again, it's worth doing what you can to improve your sleep, regardless of whether you'll need to be treated by your doctor. As you go through the programme, pay particular attention to those steps that will allow you to avoid becoming too sleepy. Also avoid caffeine and establish a balanced exercise programme.

Your doctor will treat your legs if they are significantly affecting your life. He or she may need to try several different medications, doses, or schedules before the treatment is finalized.

THE SLEEP-FITNESS LEVEL

What do you want out of life? It's not an easy question. There are many possibilities – health, excitement, service, money, and the happiness of others – but these seem to be the by-products of a successful life rather than good goals. All the attributes of good sleep – improved health, better judgement, balanced mood, better reaction time, and sharper perception – seem to contribute directly to the *character* of life:

fundamental characteristics that allow success in any task along the way. Sleep is an essential part of building, maintaining or repairing that character of life, and sleep fitness is the tool to accomplish this.

The concept of fitness as a means to improve and maintain physical activity or athleticism is a familiar one; similarly, sleep fitness will help you to get more from your sleep. You'll benefit in terms of sleep health (you'll be less likely to acquire a sleep disorder) and in terms of sleep performance (you'll sleep better, and be more prepared for the creative aspects of sleep). To accomplish this you'll need to do the right things consistently and regularly, so that you develop good habits and get better and better as you progress.

One of the best dividends from sleep fitness is the improvement that you can expect in your waking performance. We've been impressed that many studies demonstrate about a 20 per cent change for the better in a variety of tasks as a result of improved sleep. For someone in business this would mean a 20 per cent improvement in productivity, which would make a success of most companies. At home, it is harder to quantify but possible to imagine. Most people looking after small children would welcome any improvement at all. Such levels of improvement can be attained consistently and almost universally through fitter and better sleep.

Sleep fitness: how do we do it?

The backbone of your plan to attain and maintain sleep fitness will be the 'Twenty-one nights to better sleep' programme in Chapter 5. Go through it once to develop the skills that you'll need to be sleep-fit. Later you can repeat it to maintain your conditioning. Treat the sleep tips in Chapter 7 as specific exercises for particular needs. We're not asking you to become obsessed about every aspect of your sleep, but we do think that you'd benefit from dealing with even small issues as they arise.

As with any conditioning programme, the first step is to see if you're well enough to begin. We'll cover this in the next chapter.

> **Sleep fitness is probably the easiest way for most healthy people to perform better, be healthier, enjoy life more, and even live longer.**

CHAPTER 4

Checking what's wrong with your sleep

It's important to know what's wrong before we try to put it right. Many people think that they're getting good-quality sleep when, in reality, they have forgotten what it's like to wake up fully refreshed. Others believe that they don't have a sleep problem because they can fall asleep anywhere, at any time, but their friends and family tell a different story. The difficulty is that there's no simple test for sleep problems. We can't take a blood sample and measure your 'sleep level' and we can't attach electrodes to your head and know at once exactly how sleepy you are. But, after years of interviewing patients and conducting surveys in different settings, we can ask questions that give a sense of what's wrong and what you need to do about it.

We'll start with your **chief complaint**. This has been a standard feature of medicine for centuries for the simple reason that it works well. Put simply: 'What bothers you most about your sleep?' Or, 'What is bothering you in your life that you think is a result of poor sleep?' This step of the assessment is so important that it is worth writing it out before continuing. We suggest you do that here before moving on:

Lack of it

Quite often the words people use to describe their chief complaint provide clues to the next step in the assessment. Have you mentioned other health problems that are affecting your sleep, such as pain, stiffness, or headaches, for example? If so, it is quite likely that you have other medical issues in addition to your sleep problems that must also be tackled. Did you refer to a medication or treatment that has not left you entirely satisfied? This would indicate that you should consider your current medical care or relationships as well as sleep problems. Did you write about others or your environment? Again, these are issues that shouldn't be forgotten.

You may like to ask your partner or family members about your sleep. They may have a different perspective.

We can look at the specific sleep topics that you described. For most people these will be rather general and will not lead to an obvious solution. For example, the most common complaints are, 'Too tired during the day', 'Can't get to sleep at night', etc. We'll need to look into these complaints a little more deeply to understand what's going on, and there are several assessments that can help. Below is a list of some recent complaints recorded at the Sleep Disorders Center in Seattle. See whether your complaint is like any of these:

I'm tired of being tired.	I can't get to sleep because of my legs.
Snoring.	I never sleep.
Pauses in my breathing as I sleep.	I eat in my sleep.
I'm too sleepy during the day.	I'm here because of my wife.
I wake up short of breath.	I can't sleep in the same room as my partner.
I can't sleep.	Nightmares. I get night terrors.
I can't stay asleep.	I suffer from choking.
I fall asleep all the time.	I can't wake up in the morning.
I wake up screaming in the middle of the night.	

Next we'll perform a general sleep and fatigue assessment to find out how well you sleep.

HOW DO YOU SLEEP?

- Please read each question carefully, and think about your answer.
- For those with unusual sleep schedules, 'daytime' means the time that you'd normally be awake.

Have any of the following occurred over the last two weeks or so?
Mark each answer with an X. Put 'XXX' for those that occur three or more times per week.

	YES	NO
1. Have you slept for less than six hours in a 24-hour period?	XXX	
2. Have you slept for more than nine hours in a 24-hour period?		XXX
3. Have you obtained less sleep than you would have liked?	XXX	
4. Has your sleep been less restorative or refreshing than you would have liked?	XXX	
5. Have you taken more than 30 minutes to get to sleep?	XXX	
6. Have you been awake for more than 30 minutes at a time when you did not want to be?	XXX	
7. Have you woken up more than four times in your main sleep period?	X	
8. Have you needed to go to the lavatory more than twice during your main sleep period?		X
9. Have you taken more than 20 minutes to get back to sleep after you have woken up during the night?	XXX	

	YES	NO
10. Have you been sleepier during the daytime than you wanted to be?		☒
11. Have you walked in your sleep, acted out dreams, hurt yourself or others, or left the bed while you were asleep?		☒
12. Have you awakened with a snort, gasp or choke?		☒
13. Has your sleep been disturbed by pain, discomfort, etc.?		☒
14. Has your sleep been disturbed by noise, heat, light, pets, children, your partner, etc.?		☒

Most people with good sleep will have answered 'No' to all the questions on this questionnaire. This might surprise you since many of the questions seem rather innocuous. But it's hard to have good sleep fitness if you regularly have any of these problems.

If you identified several problems on this questionnaire, or if you're bothered by sleepiness, you'll almost certainly benefit from the 'Twenty-one nights to better sleep' programme in Chapter 5. Only a comprehensive programme like that one is likely to cover all the relevant issues.

If you marked only one or two items, you can start by reading the appropriate parts of Chapter 7: Sleep Tips before you begin the 'Twenty-one nights to better sleep' programme. Focus specifically on the items that you marked 'XXX', but don't ignore any of the positive items. Remember that this is not a complete list, and many other possibilities are described in this book.

A SIMPLE TEST FOR SLEEPINESS

One of the most effective tests is known as the Epworth Sleepiness Scale after the hospital in Australia where it was devised. It was originally published in the journal *Sleep*, and is reprinted here by permission. You can find the full citation in the reference section.

Filling in the grid below is the simplest way to discover whether you are sleepy.

Fill in the grid in terms of how the situations relate to you and your usual way of life recently, using the zero to three scale below. Don't count the times when you just feel tired without actually dozing off. Even if you have not done some of these things recently, try to work out how they would have affected you.

0 = would never doze
1 = slight chance of dozing
2 = moderate chance of dozing
3 = high chance of dozing

Situation	Chance of dozing
Sitting and reading	
Watching television	
Sitting still in a public place (e.g., a theatre or a meeting)	
Being a passenger in a car for an hour without a break	
Lying down to rest in the afternoon when circumstances permit	
Sitting and talking to someone	
Sitting quietly after lunch (having drunk no alcohol)	
In a car, while stopped for a few minutes in traffic	
Total score	

Your score tells us a lot about how sleepy you are. If your score is seven or less, you are an excellent candidate for the 'Twenty-one nights to better sleep' programme. If your score is 12 or more, you would benefit both from the 'Twenty-one nights to better sleep' programme and from a visit to your doctor.

If your score is between seven and 12, you'll need to consider your particular circumstances. For example, if you have a score of eleven but you know that the main problem is a young baby, the 'Twenty-one nights' programme might be appropriate. On the other hand, a score of eight with some worrying dozing when you're driving screams out for a trip to the doctor. Remember that regardless of your scores, if you feel that your sleep is dangerous or destructive to your health, you should see your doctor.

VIRGINIA MASON
SLEEPINESS ASSESSMENT

This is the latest type of assessment, which looks beyond dozing. Certainly, sleepier people do tend to doze more, but there are some people whose sleepiness is not expressed as dozing (perhaps they are just tired all the time) and others who avoid dozing (by drinking coffee, or sleeping a lot, for example). This was designed to provide a more complete assessment of sleepiness.

- Please read each question carefully, and think about your answer.
- For those with unusual sleep schedules, daytime means the time when you would normally be awake.
- Unless stated otherwise, these questions do not apply:
  - to the 30 minutes or so before your usual bedtime,
  - to times when you wake up during your main sleep period,
  - to the 15 minutes or so after you wake up in the morning.

Have any of the following occurred at least three times a week over the last two months or so?

HAVE YOU:	YES	NO
1. been sleepier than you would have liked?		✔
2. taken intentional or unintentional naps (not necessarily in bed) that have lasted for at least five minutes?		✔

HAVE YOU:	YES	NO
3. slept for more than nine hours in a 24-hour period? Include naps and time spent dozing.		☑
4. been unable to stay awake when watching television programmes or movies that interested you?		☒
5. not done things or put off doing things (e.g., family life, social activities, exercise, driving at night, work) because of sleepiness, fatigue, or lethargy?		☒
6. fallen asleep without warning, or have you been surprised to find that you had been asleep?		☒
7. tried actively to keep yourself awake or alert (e.g., by moving, singing, eating, making the room or vehicle colder, drinking caffeine)?		☒
8. made mistakes or near mistakes because of sleepiness or inattention (e.g., errors, accidents, or near accidents)?		☒
9. struggled with sleepiness when you were doing something that required your active participation (e.g., writing, driving, talking, using a computer)?		☒
10. had to stop or interrupt doing something because of sleepiness or fatigue?		☒

WOULD YOU HAVE BEEN ABLE TO:	YES	NO
11. fall asleep within 20 minutes, at any time of the day, if you were comfortable, relaxed, and undisturbed?		☒

People who do not have sleep problems answer 'No' to all the questions on the Virginia Mason Sleepiness Assessment. If you answered 'Yes' to any of these 11 questions, you would certainly benefit from taking part in the 'Twenty-one nights to better sleep' programme. If you answered

'Yes' to three or more questions, or to any of questions 7, 8, 9, or 11, you should also see your doctor.

DO YOU HAVE A SLEEP DISORDER?

If you answered 'Yes' to many of the items on the 'How do you sleep?' assessment, you may be wondering whether you have a specific sleep disorder. This is a complicated issue, but we can give some guidelines that might help.

You may have **insomnia** if:
- you routinely take more than 30 minutes to fall asleep, either at the beginning of the night or if you awaken during the night
- you're often awake earlier than you would like to be at the end of your main sleep period and you can't get back to sleep

Almost everyone who suffers from insomnia would benefit from improved sleep fitness, so we recommend proceeding with this programme. It's a good idea to go to your doctor if you are preoccupied with the problem or if it's affecting your life.

You can suspect that you don't spend enough time sleeping (**insufficient sleep syndrome**) if:
- you're always sleepy
- you wake up to an alarm clock most days of the week
- you need to 'sleep in' or nap at weekends or when you can get the chance
- you feel much less sleepy when you get more sleep, for example, at weekends or when you are on holiday

The 'Twenty-one nights to better sleep' programme is excellent for this issue. There's usually no need to see a doctor unless your sleepiness is dangerous or interfering with your life.

You might have **harmless snoring** if you snore, even loudly, and:
- you never, or only rarely, have unwelcome sleepiness
- you are certain that you don't have and have never had heart problems or high blood pressure

Follow the steps outlined in this book to overcome the social problems associated with snoring, and prevent anything more serious from developing.

You may have a medically significant breathing problem (either **sleep apnoea** or **upper airway resistance syndrome**) if some of the following apply:
- you've been told that you stop breathing for short periods when you're asleep
- you snore loudly or intermittently
- you wake up suddenly with a snort, gasp, choke, or cough
- you have unwelcome sleepiness or fatigue
- you have any of the above and heart problems or high blood pressure

See your doctor if there are obvious symptoms. Some of the suggestions in this book will help these problems, but should not be relied upon as the only course of action for what can be a severe medical problem.

Do you have **periodic limb movement disorder**?
- Does your partner complain of twitching or kicking movements of your limbs that occur while you're asleep?
- Does your sleep feel unrestful?
- Do you have unwelcome sleepiness during the day?

You may have **restless legs syndrome**, the restless, uncomfortable sensations described on page 30 if your symptoms are:
- worse in the evening or at night
- worse with immobility
- somewhat relieved by movement

If you have either of these problems, this programme can improve your sleep and may well reduce your symptoms. They often accompany other sleep disorders so it's worth visiting your doctor if your symptoms are severe.

For other sleep disorders, see your doctor.

WHAT NEXT?

Over the years we've noticed that the people who make the greatest progress in treating their sleep problems are those who are most strongly motivated. For the majority of people, just disliking something is not enough; there has to be a tangible benefit. You may like to consider some of the more common motivations and then write your own list.

Common motivations that encourage people to improve their sleep

To get rid of unwelcome sleepiness.
To feel more alert.
To sleep through the night.
To be less dangerous when driving.
To sleep in the same room as my partner.
To avoid accidents and injury.
To improve my health.
To feel better.

My motivations to improve my sleep:

Next, you should accept the magnitude of the task that faces you. Some sleep problems are the result of issues that can be resolved quickly, while others require an extended effort. So don't expect any wonder cures or overnight successes.

Finally, you'll need to recognize that the fastest way to deal with these problems is through a structured programme. This may be frustrating, because sometimes it will seem that you're addressing unimportant issues before getting down to the nitty-gritty. Let go – it works! If the solution were a simple one, you would have discovered it yourself a long time ago. Welcome to 'Twenty-one nights to better sleep'.

CHAPTER 5

Twenty-one nights to better sleep

This programme, 'Twenty-one nights to better sleep', works to improve your sleep fitness in an organized and systematic way, over a long enough period for you to see a growing improvement. Each day you will be asked to think about your habits and learn what we believe is needed for good sleep. Some of the recommendations won't apply to you, and some will go against what you would like to do. Sometimes it hurts to change things for the better. As they say, 'No pain, no gain'.

You will be asked to make many changes in these three weeks. By the end of the programme you'll be able to work out which changes were helpful, and which weren't necessary for you. We hope that you'll find the combination of changes that will help you to sleep well.

The programme is simple to follow, but you'll need to be committed to complete it, and in some cases your partner or family will need to be involved. Sometimes you may feel that you are getting worse rather than better. If you've developed bad habits as 'crutches', these will need to be removed before true improvement can occur. Remember, if the route to better sleep were easy and obvious, you would probably have discovered it for yourself a long time ago.

We expect that the programme will take you about 20 minutes a day. It will certainly help if your partner and family are supportive, so talk to them before you begin. It's particularly important that your partner understands why this is crucial for you. If you crack this problem, you'll have invested just three weeks, with the potential of a lifetime of improved sleep and all the benefits this will bring.

WHY USE THIS PROGRAMME?

There are three clear reasons for using this programme.

1. You'll learn some skills to improve your sleep.
2. You'll feel better during your waking hours.
3. You may well improve your health, and your capacity to enjoy life.

HOW THE PROGRAMME WORKS

Decide on a starting date and begin on that day. You'll tackle your poor sleep in small steps, one topic a day. Preview the material each morning even if you do most of the work later in the day. Keep a small notebook and a highlighter pen handy. **Read** the appropriate section, and **think** carefully about the advice and the actions you need to take. **Write** any decisions that you make in the box provided or your notebook, or **highlight** the relevant sentences in the text. Fill in all of the questionnaires and complete all of the exercises. Then make every effort to **accomplish** those changes. It is only through a careful and rigorous pursuit of the programme that you'll reap the right rewards.

Some people will feel immediate benefits from the changes suggested here, but it is more likely to take *at least* three weeks. You'll only learn what is important if you make adjustments slowly, and if you persist for some time. Also, sleep itself is slow to change. People can usually adjust their natural rhythms by only about an hour a day.

Although the programme is organized into daily activities, don't worry if you need more than one day to accomplish each step of the programme, and therefore more than three weeks to complete it. Just persist with it until you feel happy enough to continue. Similarly, if you have 'slipped' on an earlier issue, it is perfectly acceptable to backtrack to the relevant part and repeat the programme from that point on. All we ask is that you stay with the process (repeating the same exercises each day) and that you do not wait for your sleep or wakefulness to improve before you carry on. As we explained above, these will be some of the last changes that you notice.

How will you know if things are improving? You completed a comprehensive sleep assessment in Chapter 4, and we suggest that you repeat it at the end of the programme. In between, you'll be asked to keep track of certain key indicators each day. Please make an effort to do this every day. At the end of each week, take the time to think carefully about your progress. If you need to repeat part of the programme, do so according to the instructions. Then work through to the end.

You can also focus on one or two indicators of how well you're doing. It's best if these are to do with your wakefulness rather than being direct measures of your sleep. For example, you might pay attention to how alert you are, how well you stay awake in meetings, how troublesome driving is, or how well you're coping with life.

Of course, we can't guarantee that this programme will work for you. However, it's been successful for others, and you'll certainly learn more about your sleep and the things that help or hinder its success.

Remember: a healthy person should be capable of good, refreshing, sleep, and the bright successful wakefulness that comes from it. Good luck!

NIGHT ONE: AN ADEQUATE OPPORTUNITY FOR SLEEP

Are you allowing yourself enough time to sleep? Do you spend too much time tossing and turning? Too often these days, the pressure is on for you to be awake for as long as possible, whether for work, children, or even because of poor sleep. Let's make sure that you have the right opportunity for good-quality, consolidated sleep. Too little time means that you cannot get enough sleep. Too much means that the quality of your sleep will deteriorate as you spread your sleep too thinly.

> **You will not sleep well if you spend either too much, or too little, time in bed.**

Today you'll establish your **preferred time in bed**. This is how long you should be in bed, asleep or ready for sleep in order to get the most, best-quality sleep that you can. We'll work out how long that should be from how much time you now spend asleep or ready and available for sleep each day (your **daily opportunity for sleep**) and the total time that you're actually asleep (your **daily time spent sleeping**).

First, some calculations. (The workspace, on page 62, may be helpful.)

Time spent sleeping

How much time, on average, are you *actually asleep* each 24 hours? Add up all your hours of sleep for the last week and divide the total by seven. Include naps and dozing in front of the television, and make sure that you allow for the extra hours that you might have slept last weekend or on days when you weren't working. Don't include time that you spent in bed when you were awake. You'll find it easier to round your answer up or down to the nearest fifteen minutes.

(a) My **daily time spent sleeping** over the last week was

☐ hours, ☐ minutes.

Daily opportunity for sleep

Next, add up how much time you spend either asleep, or awake but ready for sleep. For most people this is the time that they spend in bed. Don't count time when you have no intention of being asleep (for example, when you're reading or watching television in bed). Do count time outside bed if you're asleep, dozing or trying to sleep, for example, sleeping on the sofa. Again, work out your daily average for the last week, and round your answer up or down to the nearest fifteen minutes.

(b) My **daily opportunity for sleep** over the last week was

☐ hours, ☐ minutes.

Preferred time in bed

Now you can calculate how much time you *should* be spending in bed. We say 'in bed' because in most cases it's better if you're sleeping in bed than, for example, in an armchair when watching television. There are several possibilities and you'll need to choose the one that's most appropriate for you.

- If you are often **too sleepy when you're awake but have little trouble getting to sleep**, add half an hour to your daily opportunity for sleep (b) above, to calculate your *preferred time in bed*. By 'little trouble getting to sleep' we mean that you usually spend fewer than 30 minutes trying to get to sleep. Write your preferred time in bed below (c).

- Are you **never sleepy when you are awake but do have trouble sleeping at night**? By 'trouble sleeping at night' we mean that you usually spend longer than 30 minutes trying to get to sleep at any time during the night. If so, record your preferred time in bed as half an hour *more* than your daily time spent sleeping (a). This shouldn't be less than six hours a night. If your calculated value is less than that, just record your preferred time in bed as six hours. Write your preferred time in bed below (c).

- If you're **too sleepy during the day and you have trouble sleeping in bed**, add an hour to your daily time spent sleeping (a) above, for your preferred time in bed. Write this value below (c).

- If none of these apply, stick with your current pattern!

(c) My **preferred time in bed** is

[ ] hours, [ ] minutes.

Your goal is to be in bed for your preferred time. Think about specific ways in which you will accomplish this; for example, not watching the late news, or by being in bed by 10 p.m. If there is a huge difference between your current sleep patterns and your preferred time in bed, at least commit yourself to a daily improvement of even as little as ten minutes towards your goal. If you have difficulty getting to sleep or staying asleep, it is well worth sticking to your preferred time in bed *every day*. Otherwise it's OK to sleep a little longer at weekends than during the week.

It may be helpful for you to write your conclusions in this box:

Notes or decisions about my preferred time in bed
1.
2.
3.

But...?

'I can't spend more time in bed because of my work schedule.'
We'll be discussing the answers to problems like these on a later night. For now, do what you can even by such simple methods as getting to bed earlier when you can, avoiding things that obviously conflict with more sleep (such as late television programmes), and being well organized in the hours before you go to sleep.

'I can't spend more time in bed, because I have to wait up for my spouse or children.'
Our sleep patterns are often negotiated with others, or are a compromise between our personal needs and those of the family. We will work more on this topic later, but, for now, involve others in the project, making sure that they understand how important this is to you, and how, eventually, the whole family will benefit if you get better sleep.

'I've tried this before, and it just doesn't work.'

It is difficult for people with insufficient sleep to be clear about how their sleep and wakefulness interact. After all, their system is not working, and we're sure that most of them have tried many different approaches to get better sleep. The solution is to adopt a programme that gradually assembles the building blocks for success, and allows you enough time to master each one while developing a structure that will be successful. Just changing the time they spend in bed will not guarantee perfect sleep for most people. But it is an essential part of the process.

'You just don't understand – I can't spend less time in bed because I am tired enough as it is.'

It seems paradoxical that spending less time in bed might be necessary for you to get more or better sleep, but this is a proven technique. Many people with poor sleep have gradually damaged their ability to fall into deep refreshing sleep, leaving shallow 'stretched-out' sleep that is very vulnerable to disturbance. The quickest way to restore the quality of sleep is to consolidate the sleep that does occur into a more appropriate time in bed. If the amount is not enough, the good-quality sleep can be extended gradually later on.

'I have a serious medical problem that prevents me from sleeping.'

You may still benefit from getting the right opportunity for sleep. But if your problems are too severe, this programme will have to wait. Consult your doctor or a sleep specialist.

Workspace for Night One

This table may be useful for your calculations of daily time spent sleeping:

Day	Time asleep at night (A)	Time asleep during naps, dozing, etc. (B)	Total time asleep in the 24 hours = A+B
1			
2			

Day	Time asleep at night (A)	Time asleep during naps, dozing, etc. (B)	Total time asleep in the 24 hours = A+B
3			
4			
5			
6			
7			
		TOTAL (rows 1 to 7)	
		AVERAGE	

You can use a similar table for your calculations of opportunity for sleep:

Day	Time asleep at night (A)	Time asleep during naps, dozing, etc. (B)	Total time asleep in the 24 hours = A+B
1			
2			
3			
4			
5			
6			
7			
		TOTAL (rows 1 to 7)	
		AVERAGE	

In conclusion

Today we took the first step by calculating your preferred time in bed. This will probably need to be changed as your sleep improves, and you'll return to these calculations from time to time to update it. But, for the time being, it will help to provide a solid foundation for the other changes that will follow.

NIGHT TWO: WHAT IF YOU ARE TOO SLEEPY?

Are you **too sleepy** to do things safely? Is your life a misery because of tiredness, sleepiness or fatigue? Do you make mistakes at work? You should know what to do if you find you are too sleepy to function safely.

Never do anything that risks the safety of yourself or others because you are too sleepy.

Today we'll work on sleepiness and unwelcome sleepiness. **Sleepiness** is the sensation, behaviour or consequences of sleep intruding into wakeful life. **Unwelcome sleepiness** is sleepiness that is not expected, or not wanted. We all expect to be sleepy at bedtime, or as a passenger in a car after a six-hour drive, but sleepiness at a red light after a fifteen-minute drive is *unwelcome*.

First, you need to be able to recognize unwelcome sleepiness. Do any of the following apply to you?

- **Sleep attacks:** sleep, or struggling with sleepiness, that interferes with tasks or activities in which you are an active participant.
- **Passive sleepiness:** sleep, or drowsiness, when you're relaxing or not particularly active. Do you tend to fall asleep in front of the television? In church? Reading to the children?
- **Detrimental consequences.** Regardless of how sleepy you feel, or of the other indicators of sleepiness, do you make more mistakes than you should, or drift in the lane when you're driving, or have you had accidents or near accidents? Do you put off doing things because of sleepiness?
- **Too much 'compensating' sleep.** Perhaps you compensate for sleepiness by sleeping at almost every opportunity? Do you take naps more than a couple of times a month? Do you sleep for more than eight or nine hours a night? Do you 'catch up' on your sleep every weekend? Do you sleep through alarms or need to use the snooze button?
- **Doing things to mask your sleepiness**. Sleepiness can be masked by stimulants (such as coffee). Some people mask their sleepiness by listening to loud music and standing rather than sitting.

	Midnight to 3 a.m.
Asleep, even for a moment	
Irresistible head-nodding or eye closing	
Dozing or napping	
Interrupted something that you were doing because you were too sleepy	
Didn't feel adequately alert or awake	
Mistakes, accidents, or near accidents as the result of sleepiness	
Did something (e.g., rolled down the window, or drank coffee) to combat sleepiness	
Worried, upset, or embarrassed by sleepiness	

- **You feel that you're too sleepy, or that you're worried or embarrassed about it.** Think back five or ten years: has your ability to function well during the day changed? Do others who know you well complain about your lack of energy?

Think about the last 24 hours. Mark any boxes that apply in the table above with an X. Mark 'XXX' if the situation was dangerous.

Look at the results. People with good sleep health are usually sleepy only just before (and sometimes just after) their main sleep period. Almost everybody with unwelcome sleepiness has a sleep problem, although it's possible that your sleep is poor, even though you may not feel sleepy during the daytime.

Your sleepiness may not be constant. Use the table on page 67 to see if there are particular circumstances under which your sleepiness is worse. Put an X by any circumstance under which you are ever sleepy, and mark 'XX' if you're routinely sleepy.

You may also need a 'reality check' about your sleepiness. Use the table in the workspace on page 70 to find out whether or not others think that you are as sleepy as you do.

3 a.m. to 6 a.m.	6 a.m. to 9 a.m.	9 a.m. to noon	noon to 3 p.m.	3 p.m. to 6 p.m.	6 p.m. to 9 p.m.	9 p.m. to midnight

Sleepiness is caused either by not enough sleep, or by poor-quality sleep. We're usually aware of being sleepy only when the normal things that keep us alert and awake just can't compensate. So we may feel sleepier when we're bored, or after lunch, or when we are warm; but these circumstances are really just unmasking the sleepiness that had already been there.

- Learn to recognize unwelcome sleepiness and the other ways in which you are affected by poor sleep.

CIRCUMSTANCE	SLEEPINESS
Most days	
Workdays	
Weekends	
Days following nights when I have not slept well	
Days following nights when I have used a sleeping-pill	

- Treat irresistible sleepiness under even remotely dangerous circumstances as an emergency, perhaps in the same sense that you would urgently respond to physical incapacity such as sudden vomiting. Stop whatever you are doing as soon as it is safe to do so.
- The best way to combat dangerous sleepiness is to take a nap, preferably before your sleepiness becomes dangerous.
- If you are just beginning to become sleepy, do what you can to become more alert. This might include:

  - planning a nap before it becomes too dangerous
  - becoming active; for example, moving, talking, or singing
  - avoiding boredom or monotony; for example, doing something different, talking to someone, or listening to the radio
  - cooling down: opening the windows, or turning up the air conditioning
  - seeking moderately bright light
  - eating, preferably small quantities of relatively plain food
  - drinking coffee or other caffeinated beverages. Too much caffeine should be avoided under most circumstances, particularly if you have trouble sleeping at night. But it's better to drink caffeine than to be dangerously sleepy

People respond to each of these stimuli in different ways, and what wakes up one person might make another more sleepy. Furthermore, stimulation is no good if it is too distracting. Also, it's important to realize that becoming more alert only masks sleepiness for a while, it doesn't eliminate it. Once you become too sleepy, only sleep itself will provide a lasting solution.

- If unwelcome sleepiness is at all frequent, or predictable, see your doctor.

Your goals are to be more aware of how you are during the day, and to be more responsive to sleepiness until your sleep has improved. Write your conclusions in this box:

Notes or decisions about daytime sleepiness

1.

2.

3.

But...?

'Of course I'm sleepy; I work hard.'

Yes, but even so, you might want to pay attention to your sleepiness for two reasons. First, however sleepiness is caused, it still can be detrimental to your health or well-being. You can end up paying the price for an accident, or for general lack of motivation and poor social skills, whether they result from honest labour or from a sleep problem.

Second, we often find that people with sleep disorders persist in thinking that they have no problem because it is so easy to blame their symptoms on other things, such as work. Ask yourself whether young children in the house or a tough work schedule are masking a more serious problem.

'Of course I'm sleepy, I know I have a sleep problem.'

Sleep problems often take some time to resolve, even if you are being 'aggressively' treated by a sleep specialist. In the meantime, you need to do what you can to minimize the harmful effects of unwelcome sleepiness.

'Of course I'm sleepy; I'm getting old.'

No. There's no reason why older people should be sleepy if they maintain good sleep habits and sleep health.

'I'm not sleepy; I just like resting my eyes.'

Read the descriptions of unwelcome sleepiness again. We don't care what you call it, or what you do when it happens – you'll be better off once you've dealt with it!

Workspace for Night Two

What do others think about how sleepy or alert I am?

On a scale of zero to 10, where 10 represents being as troubled by unwelcome sleepiness as you can imagine, score how sleepy you think you have been over the last two weeks.

My sleepiness score: ☐

Now ask others who know you well what score they would give you for the last two weeks.

Person	Score

In conclusion

We've covered some key points about sleepiness. You should now know how to recognize it in all its forms, and deal with it successfully. Remember, don't take chances with sleepiness and, if in doubt, see your doctor.

IN THE LAST 24 HOURS	YES	NO
Was your actual time in bed within 20 minutes of your preferred time in bed?	☐	☐

Give yourself one point for 'Yes' and no points for 'No'. Write your score in the box below, and also in the summary table on page 163.

Total points for today: ☐

If you answered 'Yes', *good!* If you answered 'No', don't be concerned, some of the other pieces of the puzzle may need to be in place before you are successful. But do try again tonight to get closer to your preferred time in bed, and also start work being less sleepy during the daytime.

NIGHT THREE: A BEDTIME THAT'S SENSIBLE FOR YOU

To get to sleep, you must be ready and able to 'let go' of wakefulness. It is not much use going to bed if you don't need to go to sleep. The time at which we are ready to go to sleep depends on how long it has been since we last slept, how alert we are, and our natural biological rhythms.

There are two key strategies to making a bedtime schedule work:

- regularity, even if your schedule is not regular (you may think that this is impossible because of young children or your work routine, but we'll show you how to achieve it),
- putting sleep into the right part of your daily biological cycle.

> **Aim for a regular bedtime at the right time for you.**

What influences the time at which you start getting ready for bed, and when you are actually ready to turn out the light? Today we'll start from your **waking-up time**, which is the final time when you wake up to begin your day. We'll calculate your **bedtime**, the time when you should get into bed. You will learn later that this is different from your **lights-out time**, the time when you are ready for sleep. The best bedtime will depend on your schedule. For example, you may do shift work, which, in this context, means any work outside the normal daytime routine of eight to ten hours within the span of 7 a.m. to 7 p.m. Remember, from your body's perspective, commuting is work.

The last week

Write down all your bedtimes for the last week. Include the occasions when you took naps at other times of the day or the night. This table may be helpful:

NIGHT	BEDTIME	NAP TIMES
1.		
2.		
3.		
4.		
5.		
6.		
7.		

Making a plan

Now draw up a plan based on your schedule, whatever that might be. You'll have to decide what best describes your routine: regular hours, an early schedule, a late schedule, working nights, or a variable or disrupted schedule. We'll deal with each possibility in turn.

Regular hours

If you have a schedule with regular hours (that is, you do more or less no work between 7 p.m. and 7 a.m. and you don't commute before 6 a.m. or after 7 p.m.), it is relatively easy to achieve a set pattern, and you should set your bedtime from the time you need to get up in the morning:

- First, decide on a comfortable time to get out of bed that will work for as many days of the week as possible. This is probably a time that allows you to get to work on time! Think about it carefully. Your first guess may be an earlier time than necessary, because you may not be preparing well the night before.

  My preferred waking-up time is ☐ a.m. / p.m.

- Next, count back the number of hours that you calculated on Night One as your preferred time in bed. This will give you the time when you need to be ready to turn out the light and start the process of falling asleep. If you want time in bed for other reasons, such as relaxing, reading, or sex, you will need to get into bed earlier.

My preferred bedtime is ☐ a.m. / p.m.

- It is really best to set this time for seven days a week and not just for workdays. Regularity is helpful, but there's no need to be inflexible. Once or twice a week these times can be delayed, i.e., made later, by up to 90 minutes, or brought forward, i.e., made earlier, by up to 30 minutes. However, on most days you should try to get to bed within 15 minutes or so of your preferred time.

If you are one of the 30 per cent of people who work between 7 p.m. and 7 a.m., or who have a disrupted schedule, setting sensible times is harder, but even more essential.

Early schedule
If you have an **early schedule**, so that you have to work before 7 a.m. or leave home for work before 6 a.m., you'll be fighting against your natural biological rhythm and it will be absolutely vital for you to keep a regular schedule. You can use the same guidelines as given above for a regular schedule to calculate your preferred times. Choose the times that would be best for you, and write them down here.

My preferred waking-up time is ☐ a.m. / p.m.

My preferred bedtime is ☐ a.m. / p.m.

Late schedule
If you have a **late schedule**, which requires you to work until the middle of the night (getting home between 11 p.m. and 3 a.m., for example):
- Go to bed as soon as you can after getting home and aim to fall asleep in 20 minutes or less.
- If you have difficulty with this, you might need to allow a suitable 'winding-down time' (perhaps 30 to 60 minutes).
- Don't leave too much to do before bed: arrange your schedule so that you can avoid eating a major meal or doing paperwork, for example.

For many people this is an easy and 'natural' schedule if:

◆   the conflict with their partner's schedule is not troublesome
◆   they can avoid trying to fit too much into each day
◆   they can wind down properly after work before trying to sleep

This is the most flexible schedule, and it doesn't much matter what time you go to sleep on your days off. Choose the times that would be best for you, and write them down here.

My preferred bedtime on workdays is [   ] a.m. / p.m.

My preferred bedtime on my days off is [   ] a.m. / p.m.

Working nights

If you **work nights**, one key concept is to keep both your main meal and some sleep time (perhaps about three hours) within the same two- to three-hour period every day, even at weekends and your days off. This regularity tends to 'anchor' your natural daily biological rhythms.

For example, perhaps you can eat your main meal at 4 or 5 p.m. on workdays, and 6 or 7 p.m. on your days off. Or always keep it around noon. You could divide your sleep in half, with the first period starting at 7 a.m. on workdays and late (3 a.m., for example) on your days off, but sticking to a second sleep period at 3 or 4 p.m. on every day of the week.

Remember the problems with circadian rhythms that were discussed on page 22? You will recall that it is easiest to get to sleep with a falling body temperature, and hardest to stay asleep when the body temperature is naturally rising in the mid- to late morning. This means that it is very difficult for someone with a normal circadian rhythm to go to bed between 6 and 9 a.m. and sleep for eight hours without interruption. For that reason, many night-workers sleep for several hours in the morning when they come home from work, and then try to sleep for a few more hours later in the day.

•   Settle on a preferred sleep zone in which you try to obtain at least three hours of sleep each day; for example, from midnight to 4 a.m.
•   Have a secondary sleep zone in which you either take a nap (if you obtained good sleep in your preferred sleep zone), or get at least

three hours of sleep (if you were disturbed in your preferred sleep zone). For example, if your preferred sleep zone is midnight to 4 a.m., your secondary sleep zone could be 2 to 6 p.m.

- Don't be afraid to take short naps (of about 20 to 30 minutes) to anticipate future sleepiness. For example, if you are due to start work at 9 p.m., you may want to take a nap at about 6 p.m.
- However, if naps interfere with your ability to get to sleep in your preferred sleep zone, you should probably reschedule them.

Choose the times that would be best for you when you are working nights, and write them down here:

My preferred sleep zone is from

[ ] a.m. / p.m. to [ ] a.m. / p.m

My secondary sleep zone is from

[ ] a.m. / p.m. to [ ] a.m. / p.m.

A variable or disrupted schedule
If you have a **variable or disrupted schedule**:

- Try to set some kind of constant pattern. For example, every day there may be three or four hours when you're more likely to be able to sleep. Give a high priority to going to bed at this preferred time, even if you are able to manage only a short while. If this sleep period can be during the night, so much the better.
- Try to 'top up' your sleep with naps at other times, so that (a) you never become really sleepy, and (b) you become used to obtaining good-quality sleep in a short time. *The usual advice about avoiding naps doesn't apply to you!* For example, if you expect to work in the late evening, but you are not sure exactly when, perhaps you could sleep for three to four hours after lunch. You might then go to bed for another 40 minutes or so in the early evening and perhaps again later if your work is delayed. Don't always expect to fall asleep when you start this routine, but by giving yourself the time in bed you will eventually learn to sleep if you need to.

Write down your preferred sleep time below, even if you will not always be able to take advantage of it:

My preferred bedtime is from

☐ a.m. / p.m. to ☐ a.m. / p.m.

Whatever routine you keep:

- Convince your partner of the seriousness of your plan. Some joint activities, including sexual intimacy, may need to be rescheduled, and you will need to respect each other's schedules.
- You will benefit from spending some time preparing for your day before you go to bed (regular and early schedules), or in the afternoon (late and night schedules).
- Get into the habit of videotaping favourite television programmes and viewing them at times that fit in with your sleep schedule. Do not alter your sleep schedule to catch your favourite programmes.

Your goal is to achieve and keep these regular schedules. Write down any thoughts about how you might accomplish this here:

Notes or decisions about my preferred bedtime and waking-up time

1.

2.

3.

But...?

'My bedtime is fixed by others in my family. I have no choice in the matter.'
First, decide whether this is truly their decision or yours. Perhaps you are influencing the overall schedule at some earlier time, by your choice of mealtime, for example. Next, discuss your preferred and actual bedtimes with your family. In many cases, some kind of

accommodation or compromise can be reached. After all, this will only be for about three weeks in the first instance.

'I will never have good sleep while I am in this job.'
You may never have perfect sleep, but your sleep can improve. Even under the most outrageous schedule you can use some of the tips given here to do better. If you eventually find that your sleep does not improve enough, you may need to consider getting a different job, but at least give yourself a chance by sticking with the programme for three weeks.

'Regardless of my good intentions, I always get to bed too late.'
This problem often results from a lack of structure earlier on. There are always many things that we would like to accomplish before going to bed, so the best chance of success is to start work on them as early as possible. Alternatively, the focus on going to bed may come too late in the sequence. Try working backward to find the point, or points, in the chain of events that will allow you to be successful. For example, your chain may be to eat dinner, feed the pets, wash the dishes, call your mother, have a bath, get undressed, clean your teeth, read a chapter or two of your book, then go to bed. In this chain, it might be necessary to have fed the pets by 7 p.m. to have a realistic chance of being in bed by 9.30 p.m. There is an exercise below that may help you to clarify and improve your chain of events.

Workspace for Night Three

Even the most disorganized people with the most outrageously disrupted schedules have some routines that influence the time leading up to bedtime. The purpose of this exercise is to enable you to understand the components of those routines, and how they fit together to make chains.

First, write down all the things that you do in the few hours before bedtime (or in the hours before you go to sleep, if you spend a long time in bed before you go to sleep). Add them to the box below, without being concerned about placement or order. Include items that occur every day, and also those that occur only once or twice a week if they are significant, but don't worry about things that happen only infrequently. We've put in a few that apply to many people, but just cross out the ones that don't apply to you.

The start of the evening	**Dinner**	**Washing-up**
Telephone calls	**Snack**	**Read**
Watch TV	**Bathroom**	**Prepare clothes for tomorrow**
Get into bed	**Go to sleep**	

Next, try to draw arrows linking the usual pathways from 'The start of the evening' to 'Go to sleep' in the order in which you normally do these things. If there are several possible orders, draw several lines.

Circle any **key links** in this chain other than 'The start of the evening' and 'Go to sleep'. By 'key', we mean events that have to be completed by a certain time if you are to get to sleep on time. For example, you might know that you won't be asleep on time if you're not in the bathroom by 9:45 p.m. It's usually helpful to have one or two key links.

Use the table overleaf to design an ideal evening that would allow you to get everything done, and to be in bed on time. There is space for three chains. Use these for different nights or perhaps different variations of your ideal schedule. You need only put in times for the key links, unless you feel other times would be helpful.

Chain 1		Chain 2		Chain 3	
Event	Time	Event	Time	Event	Time
The start		The start		The start	
Go to sleep		Go to sleep		Go to sleep	

Once you're happy with this schedule, use it to guide your evenings, and see if you really can get to bed on time.

In conclusion

Over the last three days we've established your preferred time in bed, and your preferred bedtime. These lay a solid foundation for the timing of your sleep. It's worth investing the effort to use these times on a regular basis, and the daily assessments should help to tell you how well you are doing.

IN THE LAST 24 HOURS	YES	NO
Was your actual time in bed within 20 minutes of your preferred time in bed?	▢	▢
Were you ever inappropriately sleepy?	▢	▢

Count up the points you have scored. Each tick in a shaded square scores one point. Then write your total points for the day in the box below, and also in the summary table on page 163.

Total points for today:

If you scored one or two points, *good!* As you have seen today, there are many elements of good sleep health that need to be in place before you can start being successful. Even if you didn't score a single point, go on to Night Four. As we discussed above, if you are dangerously sleepy, you should avoid dangerous situations until your sleeping problems have been resolved.

NIGHT FOUR: MAKING THE BEST USE OF COFFEE, TEA AND SOFT DRINKS

Today we'll review your use of **stimulants**, (substances which promote alertness) and especially caffeine (a type of stimulant which interferes with a particular neurotransmitter, adenosine, in the brain).

Caffeine

Many people talk about having a cup of coffee to wake them up or to get them going, but few realize that caffeine, under some circumstances, can increase sleepiness. So should you drink caffeine, and if so, when? Caffeine is a potent alerting substance that can mask all kinds of sleepiness, but unfortunately there are four drawbacks.

- Overuse reduces effectiveness, so that the effect you expect may not be there when you need it.
- The alerting effect lasts for a very long time and can interfere with sleep long after you think that it's gone.
- Caffeine can increase anxiety, which can disrupt sleep.
- Drinking too much caffeine can actually make you sleepier, rather than more alert.

Other stimulants can also counteract sleepiness, but on the other hand can lead to poor sleep, anxiety, and even heart problems. Therefore, stimulants, including coffee and tea, need to be used strategically and carefully. You need to be aware of how much you have drunk, and the effect that it has had on you.

> **Caffeine: a moderate amount, taken early and in one go, is most effective.**

How many caffeinated beverages do you drink? This includes not only coffee but colas and other caffeinated carbonated beverages, teas, and cocoa, medications with caffeine in them (read the small print), and chocolate-covered coffee beans, etc.

- Plan, and ration, your caffeine intake. The more sparingly it's used, the more effective it is. Aim for the equivalent of three cups or fewer a day.
- Caffeine can make your sleep less refreshing, even if you don't realize it. Avoid drinking caffeine within *ten hours* of bedtime, unless you need to drink it to keep you alert enough to avoid accidents or other problems with sleepiness.
- Caffeine only *masks* sleepiness, it doesn't really get rid of it. If you have to drink caffeine to keep yourself safely alert, you should see your doctor.
- Too much caffeine can actually make you feel sleepier rather than more alert. This is partly because of disturbance to your night's sleep, and partly through interference with neurotransmitters in your brain. As few as six cups a day can do this.
- If you drink coffee or tea at work to keep yourself alert, it will be most effective if you drink most of it at the beginning of your shift or day, and less thereafter. You may be more sleepy drinking six cups spread evenly through your shift than having two cups at the start, with perhaps a third and final cup after another hour and then nothing more.
- Develop a routine, with each cup of coffee or tea having a special place in your schedule.
- Develop alternatives to the habit. Try walking around, or drinking water or juice when you might have been having one too many coffees.
- Try to have one day a week without coffee, or where you drink considerably less than usual. This will improve the effectiveness of coffee during the rest of the week. If you get headaches on your coffee-free day, you have been drinking too much coffee.
- If you're using caffeine to combat sleepiness (when you are driving, for example), remember that it can take up to 20 minutes to take effect. In the meantime, get some exercise and fresh air, or, preferably, if it is safe to do so, take a short nap.

Nicotine

Nicotine both stimulates and relaxes, but is not consistently useful in aiding alertness. If you smoke:

- Consider whether now might be a good time to give up smoking as part of your attempt to improve the quality of your sleep.
- Never smoke in bed, or if you wake up during the night. The nicotine will disrupt your sleep, and, apart from anything else, the risk of dropping a lighted cigarette and setting fire to the bed or house is just too great.
- Try to increase the time between cigarettes, preferably by at least half as much again. So if you are a one-pack-a-day smoker, try to go from one cigarette every 45 minutes to one every one and a quarter hours.
- Seek out alternatives to the places or situations that encourage you to smoke the most. If your spouse smokes, perhaps you can agree to make the house and car, or even just the bedroom, smoke-free zones.

Another consideration, if you are using nicotine or drinking too much caffeine, is whether your **overall nutrition** is good. Are you also eating too much convenience or junk food, or missing meals? You'll find that a balanced diet is helpful in the context of rebalancing your life, and that good nutrition certainly promotes good sleep.

Your goal is to use stimulants wisely and be aware of the effect that they have on you.

Notes or decisions about the stimulants that I use

1.

2.

3.

But…?

'I can't drink less coffee – I'm sleepy enough as it is.'
This attitude is understandable enough, but there are several reasons (given above) why more caffeine is not the solution. Caffeine masks sleepiness and may be disrupting your sleep. For the duration of this programme, try to comply with these guidelines strictly unless to do so

is likely to be dangerous, in which case see your doctor.

'I don't need to change my coffee-drinking habits because caffeine doesn't affect me.'
Many people do not feel that caffeine disturbs their sleep, and believe that they can drink caffeine late at night without penalty. Often, this is because the person is already somewhat sleep-deprived, with a sleep debt that overcomes the effect of the caffeine. When you are trying to improve your sleep health, too much caffeine will almost always complicate your progress. So, for the duration of this programme, keep within the guidelines.

'I've tried to give up smoking so many times that I know that any further attempt is just a waste of time.'
Maybe so, but now you have one more reason, on top of the many health and survival reasons that you have heard in the past. Obviously, we would encourage you to seek the help and tools that you need to quit for good. But, even if now is not the right time, look carefully at the suggestions given above that will minimize the impact of nicotine on your sleep whether you give up smoking or not.

Workspace for Night Four

Use the following table to calculate your daily stimulant use. We've indicated the average effect from a variety of drinks and some foods. In most blocks you can see three values for weak, average (in bold) and strong. The values are based on a 'recommended' maximum of 100 units per day. Count the number of uses in a typical day, and multiply by the most appropriate strength. Add up all your values for the grand total of the day.

COFFEE	Per 100ml	Amount	Cup 200ml	Amount	Mug 300ml	Amount
Filter	17-**32**-51		34-**64**-102		51-**96**-153	
Instant	8-**18**-34		16-**36**-68		24-**54**-102	
Decaffeinated	0-1-2		0-2-4		0-3-6	
ESPRESSO	Single	Amount	Double	Amount		
	33		58			
TEA	Per 100ml	Amount	Cup 200ml	Amount	Mug 300ml	Amount
	8-**18**-32		16-**36**-64		24-**54**-96	
ICED TEAS	Per 100ml	Amount	Glass 350ml	Amount		
	9		32			
COCOA	Per 100ml	Amount	Cup 200ml	Amount	Mug 300ml	Amount
	7-**9**-13		14-**18**-26		21-**27**-39	
SOFT DRINKS	Per 100ml	Amount	Can 354ml	Amount	Large	Amount
	4-6		15-20		30-40	
CHOCOLATE	Per 100g	Amount	Bar	Amount		
	22		28			
ALERTNESS PILLS	Per pill	Amount				
	42-125					
PAIN KILLERS	Per pill	Amount				
	0-**17**-27					
GRAND TOTAL						

Most people will do well with a daily value of 100 or less, especially if used more than ten hours before bedtime. If you are having trouble getting to sleep, try for a value as close to zero as you can. Robust sleepers can often consume 200 units without recognizing an effect, although some influence on your sleep or wakefulness is likely to be occurring.

In conclusion

The quality of your sleep is worth some effort. We hope you've learnt that you'll get the greatest benefit from stimulants if you are careful about how much you drink and when. We'll return to the subject of timing (see page 97) after we've tackled the most important topic: rebalancing your life.

IN THE LAST 24 HOURS	YES	NO
Was your actual time in bed within 20 minutes of your preferred time in bed?	▨	☐
Were you ever inappropriately sleepy?	☐	▨
Was your actual bedtime within 30 minutes of your preferred bedtime?	▨	☐

Count the number of ticks or crosses in the shaded squares. Each one scores one point. Then write your total points for the day in the box below, and also in the summary table on page 163.

Total points for today: ☐

If you scored two or three points, *good!* If you did not score any points, look carefully for the reasons. If you feel you are making progress on all of the items in each area (even if you didn't answer these questions correctly), proceed to Day Five. If not, or if you are not really sure about any of these, you might be better off restarting the programme. It will only add a night or two to the three weeks, but will significantly improve your chance of success.

As always, if you are dangerously sleepy, you should avoid risky situations until your sleeping problems have been resolved.

NIGHT FIVE: REBALANCING YOUR LIFE

Just as you can't function well during the day if you have poor sleep, it is also harder to sleep well if your waking life is out of balance. The daily stresses and strains of dealing with work, family problems, or money, for example, need to be balanced by some waking distractions and pleasures such as hobbies, crafts, or sports.

This is difficult, because time is short for most of us; and for people with poor sleep the motivation for doing something else is often lacking.

> **Each week, spend at least half an hour doing activities that are: physically active; pure fun; just for yourself; charitable or just for others, and peaceful or spiritual.**

Today we'll provide some tools for you to assess the balance of your life, and to rebalance it if necessary. This is essential if you are to get the best sleep, and to get the most from your sleep. It will involve a degree of **letting go**, the process of determining that a current course of action is not in one's best interests, and then actually changing to a better plan.

- Think about the kinds of things you have done in the last two weeks in the following categories:
  - physical effort
  - exercise
  - relaxation away from home
  - time purely for yourself
  - something fun
  - quality time with your partner or friends
  - something charitable or spiritual

- Are there any gaps? If so, plan some time in each of these categories. Choose the simplest, most enjoyable options. If you haven't had time for such activities in the past, elaborate or complex plans are unlikely to succeed.
- It's better if some of the activities are regular commitments, preferably with friends. This may encourage you to keep up with

the new activities.

- To make time for these new activities, eliminate some things that you consider to be 'low-return', for example, marginally interesting television programmes, or long phone calls. This may require some new discipline, and some letting go.
- You'll have to consider the needs of your partner or family. See if there are changes to your schedule that might benefit them, so that it is easier for them to give their support. For example, it might be easier for your family to accept a new activity that takes you out of the home if you are also more committed to some activities which mean a lot to them. One example might be to take your children swimming or cycling.
- Don't try to overdo things, though. If you overcommit yourself for the first week, the chances are that you'll get frustrated when other obligations arise. Be realistic, and enjoy yourself.

Your goal is to reach a point where you have several different meaningful activities in your life that can balance and support each other.

Notes or decisions about rebalancing my life

1.

2.

3.

But…?

'I don't have enough time to do anything else.'

There are two answers to this. First, if you really do not have enough time to balance your life, you are in deep trouble! Your sleep and eventually your overall health will suffer. Second, there are ways to accomplish this balance without using up yet more time. Some of the things you do already can be made more useful. For example, try to go for a walk with a colleague instead of working through lunch, take the stairs instead of the lift, or have some quiet time while weeding the garden.

'How can I do anything else when I'm feeling this sleepy?'
If you are so sleepy, tired, or fatigued that you cannot balance your life, you almost certainly have a medical problem that requires attention. Why not make the first step of the process a visit to your family doctor for a thorough check-up?

Workspace for Night Five

Use this chart to list the activities you do in each of the five major categories and plan others that will lead to a balanced life.

	THINGS I DO NOW	THINGS I COULD DO
Exercise		
Pure fun		
Just for myself		
Charitable, or just for others		
Peaceful, spiritual, or renewing		

In conclusion

A single change towards a more balanced life might be one of the most important things that you do for your sleep health.

IN THE LAST 24 HOURS	YES	NO
Was your actual time in bed within 20 minutes of your preferred time in bed?	■	☐
Were you ever inappropriately sleepy?	☐	■
Was your actual bedtime within 30 minutes of your preferred bedtime?	■	☐
Did you drink caffeine within 10 hours of bedtime?	☐	■
Are you a non-smoker, a smoker who did not smoke, or, if you are a smoker, did you increase the average time between cigarettes by more than five minutes?	■	☐

Count the ticks or crosses in the shaded squares. Each scores one point. Then write your total points for the day in the box below, and also in the summary table on page 163.

Total points for today: ☐

If you scored three or more points, *good!* If you scored one or two points but you're still making good progress, proceed to Day Six. Otherwise repeat the most relevant topics.

NIGHT SIX: NAPPING

A nap is any short sleep episode that occurs outside your main sleep period. It supplements your primary sleep. Naps may be planned (for example, going to bed for an hour after lunch) or unplanned (dozing in front of the television).

- On the plus side, napping can be very refreshing and restore alertness.
- But it can be damaging if it prevents you from being sleepy enough at bedtime to obtain deep, refreshing, well-consolidated sleep in your main sleep period.

After short naps (about 20 or 30 minutes), you can wake up refreshed. Longer naps may involve deeper stages of sleep and leave you groggy when you wake up. Very long naps have all the characteristics of shortened regular sleep and should, on the whole, be avoided by people with a regular sleep schedule.

> **Take a nap if you are dangerously sleepy, or if you do not have a regular schedule.**

When do you nap, or doze? At what times of day could you nap if you were comfortable and undisturbed?

Take a short nap whenever you're dangerously sleepy. Make sure that you can do this safely. If you're driving, try to anticipate sleepiness and stop at a busy rest area. Lock your doors and windows. On longer trips, consider stopping at a hotel or motel and resting overnight. If you have unwelcome sleepiness you should avoid the activities in which it occurs and talk to your doctor about it.

While you're working, you should nap only when you're dangerously sleepy. You are dangerously sleepy if:
- you have an irresistible urge to sleep, with head-nodding or eye-closing, or a struggle to maintain your focus or concentration, *and*
- this is not promptly resolved by actions to combat monotony or boredom (cooling down, talking to someone, eating or drinking, etc.).

These circumstances call for a short emergency nap, if that can be achieved safely. You should treat them in the same way as a sudden illness, and you should seek medical attention if they happen without an obvious explanation.

After you have been napping, you should allow five to 10 minutes to overcome the grogginess that sometimes accompanies awakening before you need to make important decisions or judgements.

- If you have a regular schedule with most of your sleep at night, and you have been following the advice given so far, naps should be needed extremely rarely, and you should know why you need one. Mostly they should occur when you have been forced out of your regular routine, for example, when you have been travelling, or if you have had an early meeting or a late social event, or if you've been ill.
- Naps are sensible if you have any kind of variable or disrupted schedule, or don't obtain most of your sleep at night. They may even be extended into a split sleep schedule.
- Avoid napping if it interferes with your main sleep period unless to do so would leave you dangerously sleepy.

More information on the positive use of napping is given on pages 167 and 229.

Your goal is to manage your sleep and wakefulness to avoid or minimize unwelcome sleepiness.

Notes or decisions about my need for naps
1.
2.
3.

But…?

'Even though I am too tired to function properly, I can never nap.'

Ask yourself why you have difficulty falling asleep for a nap. If you have a physical problem (such as pain) which interferes with sleep, it might be worth going back to your doctor about the problem. If you have trouble getting to sleep for a nap on some occasions but not others, consider the circumstances and timing of your nap attempts. Some people have difficulty sleeping in unsafe or stressful situations; others have predictable difficulty sleeping at the 'wrong' part of their daily cycle. But perhaps your difficulty getting to sleep is just another manifestation of an insomnia problem. If your life is being compromised by poor sleep, persist with this programme and, if necessary, seek professional help.

'I'd love to nap, and I'd be a whole lot safer, but my company does not allow napping on work premises.'

This is a difficult one. Almost certainly your company expects you to be ready for work in every way, and this includes being capable of being fully alert for the entire time that you are on their premises. For your part, you can try to be conscientious in following the suggestions in this book. However, for any number of reasons, you may still be less than ideally alert, and would feel safer napping. First, establish whether you have a sleep disorder that requires medical attention. Next, check with your company about the policy, and whether there are plans to modify it in the light of recent attention to the dangers of sleepiness in the workplace.

Workspace for Night Six

How much time do you spend napping? Write down situations under which:

you are likely to take a nap

napping or dozing makes you feel better

napping or dozing stop you feeling sleepy for a couple of hours or more

napping or dozing interfere with your night's sleep

IN THE LAST 24 HOURS	YES	NO
Was your actual time in bed within 20 minutes of your preferred time in bed?	▨	☐
Were you ever inappropriately sleepy?	☐	▨
Was your actual bedtime within 30 minutes of your preferred bedtime?	▨	☐
Did you drink caffeine within 10 hours of bedtime?	☐	▨
Are you a non-smoker, a smoker who did not smoke or, if you are a smoker, did you increase the average time between cigarettes by more than five minutes?	▨	☐
Did you do any of the activities from Night Five (exercise, something fun, something for yourself, something charitable or for others, something peaceful or spiritual)?	▨	☐

Count the number of ticks or crosses in the shaded squares to find your total points for the day. Write your score in the box below, and also in the summary table on page 163.

Total points for today: ☐

In conclusion
Congratulations! You are a third of the way through the programme. Tomorrow we'll assess how you're doing.

NIGHT SEVEN: HOW ARE YOU DOING?

It's time to review your progress. It's probably too early for there to have been any dramatic or noticeable changes to your sleep, although some of the foundations for good sleep health should be in place. Now is the time to decide whether you would benefit from more work on some of the earlier topics, or whether you can move on. If in doubt, it is better to repeat sections than to proceed too quickly. You can use the extra columns on the summary sheet on page 163 if necessary.

How well is the programme going?

You've been monitoring your progress on a daily basis by answering questions about the previous days, and writing your daily scores on the summary sheet. Now count up your total points for the questions under 'In the last 24 hours' for the last six nights. Enter this total in the box labelled 'first week total' on the summary sheet. If you've repeated any sections, count only your most recent points. In other words, count one score for each of the six nights. There is a possible maximum of 17 points.

- If you scored more than 10, you're doing well.
- If you scored between six and 10, you're making progress, but there are some issues which require some further persistence.
- If you scored less than six you should review some of the earlier sections. Find the earliest one that gave you problems and restart from that point. Don't worry about spending two or three days on topics you find particularly difficult if you have to.

What kind of effect is it having on your sleep health?

We can assess your sleep health by how alert you are during your waking hours, and by how restful your main sleep period is. Remember that it may be too early for a large improvement.

Answer the following questions by indicating the number of days or nights in the last week on which the following have occurred. Your answer should be between zero and six for each question.

ON HOW MANY DAYS OR NIGHTS	NUMBER (0-6)
Did it take you more than 20 minutes to fall asleep?	
Were you awake for more than one hour in your main sleep period?	
Did you wake up more than five times in your main sleep period?	
Were you dangerously sleepy (see page 91)	
Were you sleepier than you would have liked to have been?	
TOTAL	

Write your total score on the summary sheet (page 164) in the 'Sleep health scores' chart, in the box marked 'Week One'. It will provide a record of your progress through the programme and this score should decrease as you make more progress.

Fine-tuning your preferred time in bed

It's possible that by now you'll need to adjust your preferred time in bed. This will almost certainly be the case if you are still sleepy during the daytime, or if you are still having difficulty getting to sleep or staying asleep. Go back to Night One (page 59) to see if an adjustment needs to be made.

> **Notes or decisions about my progress so far**
>
> 1.
>
> 2.
>
> 3.

Workspace for Night Seven

Let's keep track of the work so far. How many sections have been:

	Night(s)
helpful?	
unnecessary?	
unhelpful?	

In conclusion

We've tackled many of the issues that concern the timing of your sleep, and now we'll be covering more topics that improve its quality. Remember **persistence,** the ability to keep going in order to reach a goal.

NIGHT EIGHT: REORGANIZING YOUR BEDROOM

The old claim that we spend a third of our lives in bed is true, so a little concern about the bedroom is in order. The bedroom influences our sleep in several ways. The physical environment is important while we sleep, and many people have disturbed sleep because they are too hot, cold, uncomfortable, or are disturbed by noise, often without being fully aware of the reason. But the psychological environment may be as or more important, as far as getting to sleep is concerned.

> **Reserve the bedroom for sleep, intimacy, and such 'comfort' activities as getting dressed.**

Today we'll work on a bedroom that is **tranquil**: free from mental agitation, disturbance or turmoil.

- What can you see in your bedroom that has nothing to do with sleep, relaxation, or 'comfort' activities, such as getting dressed?
- Remove anything that does not belong in the bedroom, especially:
  - anything that turns the bedroom into an office (e.g., desks and computers)
  - the television
  - work or hobby tools
  - items being stored (unless truly out of sight)
  - junk.

- We've found very little evidence to show that books are a problem, so we're not about to deny you your bedtime reading. Radios are not a problem either, unless you habitually fall asleep with the radio on.
- Televisions are an interesting case. While they are often used for relaxation, and it seems easy enough to fall asleep in front of the television, watching television in bed does interfere with good sleep. To avoid this problem, move the television from the bedroom. If you can, set up a viewing place elsewhere in the house that is comfortable and relaxing.

- Make changes, even small ones, that make your room more comfortable. These might include adjusting the lighting, changing the curtains or blinds, adjusting the temperature, or being tidier.
- Make sure that the bedroom is the right temperature. Several studies indicate that a colder bedroom, where the temperature is about 16°C (65°F), produces the best sleep. However, have plenty of warm covers: you shouldn't feel cold, although you shouldn't be waking up in a sweat either.
- Don't be fooled into thinking that an over-firm mattress is appropriate. Comfortable support is what matters. If you think your mattress may be bothering your sleep, try sleeping somewhere else in the house (even on the sofa), or preferably in a hotel, and see what difference it makes.
- When dealing with noise, remember that it is often the difference between a loud noise and the background noise that causes most problems. For this reason, surprising though it might seem, some people sleep better with background noise, and prefer to have a fan or 'white-noise' machine on. If you are a shift-worker, it is probably a good idea to have some earplugs handy for those days when you feel particularly sensitive to noise or the rest of your family is finding it hard to keep quiet.
- If you sleep on several pillows, or sleep better in a propped position, try to work out why. If it is because of breathing problems or heartburn, you would probably do better if you put four- to six-inch blocks under the legs at the head of your bed. This will stop your body being bent as you sleep, which, incidentally, exacerbates both apnoea (pauses in breathing as you sleep) and reflux (acid coming up from your stomach and causing heartburn or an acid taste).
- Avoid being disturbed by light when you sleep. This is especially important if you are a shift-worker who is trying to sleep during the day. Many people find that they sleep best in complete darkness (which can be achieved by placing cardboard over the window, using blackout fabric, or sleeping in a basement), while others find this somewhat disorienting and may wake up feeling groggy. One solution is to buy and use a dawn-simulator, which

gradually increases the light intensity of some bright bedside lamps in a way that simulates natural dawn. If you're a shift-worker, or if you need to nap when you travel, it might be worthwhile having some eye-shades.

- If you want to go to sleep while your partner is reading, you should either negotiate for him or her to go elsewhere, or invest in a small light (perhaps even the directed-beam kind that clips to a book) so that you can remain relatively undisturbed.

Your goal is to create a restful, pleasant sleeping environment.

Notes or decisions about my bedroom

1.

2.

3.

But...?

'I don't have the money to change my bedroom now.'

This is not about money. It is about making what we have suitable for our needs (we're sure the people with the most luxurious bedrooms do not sleep any better). Tidying, cleaning, and changing priorities are all cheap. Leave until last any decisions about your mattress – the only significant expense that it is difficult to avoid – and plan your purchase carefully. Advice on mattresses is given on page 186.

'My partner likes to have the television and rowing-machine in our bedroom. What can I do?'

Get a new partner! If that isn't practical, first spend some time establishing how important your sleep is to each of you. Try the other things that we suggest, and then talk to your partner about your needs and these suggestions. Make the discussion focus on what can be done to help your sleep, not on what he or she can do with the rowing-machine.

Workspace for Night Eight

List the three worst things about your bedroom and what you could do about them.

1.	
2.	
3.	

Ask your partner to do the same.

1.	
2.	
3.	

Does this lead to any additional insight? Does it give you a sense of priority or common ground about what should be changed?

In conclusion

You may not have accomplished everything that you planned to do with your bedroom today, but don't forget about it. Persist with those minor changes until you feel satisfied that your sleeping environment will not stand in the way of good sleep.

IN THE LAST 24 HOURS	YES	NO
Was your actual time in bed within 20 minutes of your preferred time in bed?	▨	☐
Were you ever inappropriately sleepy?	☐	▨
Was your actual bedtime within 30 minutes of your preferred bedtime?	▨	☐
Did you drink caffeine within 10 hours of bedtime?	☐	▨
Are you a non-smoker, a smoker who did not smoke, or, if you are a smoker, did you increase the average time between cigarettes by more than five minutes?	▨	☐
Did you do any of the activities from Night Five (exercise, something fun, something for yourself, something charitable or for others, something peaceful or spiritual)?	▨	☐
Did you work at night, in the evening, or the early morning and take a nap?	▨	☐
Did you sleep at night and also take a nap during the day?	☐	▨

Count the number of ticks or crosses in the shaded squares to find your total points for the day. Write your score in the box below, and also in the summary table on page 163.

Total points for today:

NIGHT NINE: A BETTER BEDTIME ROUTINE

The hours before bedtime and what you do in them play an important part in getting to sleep easily, and in the quality of your night's sleep. Generally, sleep is easier if you are well relaxed, your body temperature is dropping, and you have a regular routine so that the physiological preparations for sleep are harmonized.

> **Do only relaxing activities (and don't watch television) in the half-hour before sleep.**

Your bedtime routine is the sequence of things that you do as you get ready to go to bed. On Night Three we looked at the contribution of the bedtime routine towards getting to bed on time. Now we're interested in it from the perspective of **relaxation**, the diminution of tension. Before we fall asleep we need relaxed muscles, a lower brain temperature, and mental peacefulness.

- In the two hours before bedtime, avoid activities that will stir you up: exercise, eating (other than light snacks), work, worry, arguments, and discussions.
- *Before you start your bedtime routine*, think ahead! If you prepare your clothes, food, or the things that you'll need during the next workday you may be able to sleep-in a little longer, and go to sleep slightly less anxious about the day ahead.
- Do disrupting activities or chores earlier in the evening: make a point of getting them out of the way at least an hour before bedtime. This should probably include telephone calls, especially duty or business calls.
- Time your bedtime routine so that you avoid eating a meal or drinking alcohol in the three hours before bedtime. Digestion increases your metabolic rate and the blood flow to the gastrointestinal tract for at least an hour or so, which counters the natural slowing down that is necessary for falling asleep. This is much less of a problem if you eat only small quantities of easily digestible food, for example, a few plain biscuits or a banana.

- Avoid telephone calls within an hour or so of bedtime. For now, tell callers that you're participating in this programme and would prefer calls at other times of the day. Telling late callers that you were getting ready to go to bed may be sufficient to change their calling habits. Alternatively, simply switch on an answering machine at these times.
- Avoid discussing work or family problems (particularly finances), in the hour or so before you fall asleep, and especially when you're in bed. This may require reaching an agreement with your partner. You may want to arrange a specific time to follow up on these issues, so that you are not just avoiding things that need to be discussed.
- Falling asleep with the light or radio on conditions you to a specific stimulus. This is not helpful, and may cause you problems.
- Some people find that a warm bath or shower improves the bedtime routine. This works because it is mentally and physically relaxing, and the rapid drop in body temperature afterwards is conducive to sleep. Make sure that the water is not too hot, since that can raise your body temperature too much and prevent sleep until it cools.
- Remember to use the bedroom only for sleep, intimacy, or quiet pleasures such as reading
- Write down your usual bedtime routine, and also what you think an ideal routine would be. What prevents you from having an ideal routine now?

Television
Don't watch television in bed in the hour or so before you go to sleep.

- The programmes may be alerting or disturbing, even if you don't realize that they are affecting you.
- Watching television modifies your bedtime: you're more likely to stay awake until the end of a programme, and perhaps even begin watching the next to see what it's like.
- You may be conditioning yourself to the wrong associations, either associating the bedroom with waking activities, or associating falling asleep with a powerful stimulus (the television), which will then restrict your ability to fall asleep, or to sleep well, when the

television is switched off. You may well get into the bad habit of falling asleep with the television on, only to be awakened if your partner turns it off.

Even watching television outside the bedroom as part of the bedtime routine can cause problems. Many people watch the news and then go to bed, unaware of the physiological arousal or disturbance that has been caused.

If you feel that it is difficult to put a buffer of 30 to 60 minutes between watching television and going to sleep, try not watching within an hour of bedtime for a couple of weeks and see what difference it makes.

Your goal is to have a bedtime routine that feels relaxing and leaves you ready for sleep at bedtime on at least 10 days in every two weeks.

Notes or decisions about my bedtime routine

1.

2.

3.

But…?

'I work until midnight. I have to eat and rush to bed otherwise I just won't get enough sleep.'

True. But you can do some things to minimize this problem. First, you can do some advance preparation before you go to work. Next, try to have a meal break at work where you eat a substantial meal, so that you need only have a light snack when you get home. Finally, start some of the relaxation process before you leave work. You could at least stop drinking coffee, and make some plans for the next day. In short, try to leave as little to do as possible for those precious minutes between getting home and getting between the sheets.

'We like watching television in bed.'
And that is fine if you don't have a sleep problem, and don't ever acquire a sleep problem. Watching television in bed as part of your sleep routine will almost certainly lead to difficulties at one time or another. For one week try not watching television in bed and see what difference it makes. Or restrict your bedtime viewing to one or two nights a week.

Workspace for Night Nine

1. Repeat the exercises from Night Three (page 71) now that you are changing some of the things you do before bedtime. Are there any changes in the timing of your bedtime routine?

2. Make a list of the people who have a habit of calling you too late at night. Practise what you should say to them to improve this situation. If necessary, tell them that you are involved in this sleep programme and shouldn't be disturbed after, say, 7 p.m.

In conclusion
It shouldn't have taken you long to work out a good bedtime routine, but the difficulty will be maintaining it. That's one of the advantages of a timed programme like this. With a good bedtime routine your body and brain should be more ready for sleep when you get into bed.

IN THE LAST 24 HOURS	YES	NO
Was your actual time in bed within 20 minutes of your preferred time in bed?	�	☐
Were you ever inappropriately sleepy?	☐	▪
Was your actual bedtime within 30 minutes of your preferred bedtime?	▪	☐
Did you drink caffeine within 10 hours of bedtime?	☐	▪
Are you a non-smoker, a smoker who did not smoke or, if you are a smoker, did you increase the average time between cigarettes by more than five minutes?	▪	☐
Did you do any of the activities from Night Five (exercise, something fun, something for yourself, something charitable or for others, something peaceful or spiritual)?	▪	☐
Did you work at night, in the evening, or the early morning and take a nap?	▪	☐
Did you sleep at night and also take a nap during the day?	☐	▪
Were you satisfied with the comfort, light, heat, and noise in your bedroom?	▪	☐

Count the number of ticks or crosses in the shaded squares to find your total points for the day. Write your score in the box below, and also in the summary table on page 163.

Total points for today: ☐

You should have scored five or more points. If you scored fewer, go back and repeat any sections that you find consistently difficult.

NIGHT TEN: GETTING TO SLEEP

If you're in bed and sleep is not imminent, you may be training yourself to develop even worse sleep. Also, you may become frustrated, upset, or angry, which will make sleep even less likely. In a single night we cannot deal with all the problems that have allowed insomnia to develop, probably over years. But we can make a start on the issues that are perpetuating it or making it worse. Even if you fall asleep easily, it is worth paying attention to this night of the programme. Sooner or later almost everyone suffers from insomnia.

Get out of bed after a reasonable time if sleep is not imminent.

We can't possibly cover the whole topic of insomnia in one session, so we'll focus on the inadvertent habits that tend to perpetuate poor sleep and make it worse. We'll use some **sleep restriction therapy** (a special technique) and some other ideas to tackle **conditioning** (an inadvertent development of a response [such as frustration] to a condition [sleeplessness] which then perpetuates the condition) to avoid **frustration** (a sense of insecurity, discouragement and dissatisfaction arising from thwarted desires).

- Do you ever lie in bed trying to get to sleep? Which of the following apply to you: racing brain, worry, frustration, anger, or can't switch off? Does this sensation relate to sleep or some other problem?
- Hide your clock, or at least, turn the face so that you can't see the time during the night. Clock-watching can increase frustration.
- Sometimes getting out of bed until you begin to feel sleepy enough for sleep is a good way of breaking the cycle. As a general rule, you should get out of bed whenever you become frustrated about sleeping difficulties, and also if you have been awake for 30 minutes or more at the start of the night, or for about 10 minutes during the night and sleep is not imminent. Again, don't watch the clock to do this. Just get out of bed if sleep is becoming less rather than more likely.

- When you get up, keep yourself warm and comfortable. You should try to do something that is relaxing but involves no risk of your falling asleep before you can get back into bed. Be wary about watching television: it can be stimulating or frustrating, and it may distract you from becoming gradually more relaxed. It may also turn into a habit, encouraging you to wake up more fully if you stir during the night. Reading, or drinking a warm, caffeine-free beverage, are better options.
- When you feel sleepy, get back into bed, but don't expect that sleep will come at once. You may have been conditioning yourself against sleep for some time and it will take more than one night to re-condition.
- Some people derive benefit from relaxation tapes or relaxation exercises when they are trying to get to sleep. Others find them irritating and distracting. These topics are dealt with in more detail on page 221.
- Some awakening, especially early-morning awakening (i.e., waking up too early and being unable to get back to sleep) may be the result of another problem, such as depression or menopause. If this is a regular problem, and is not happening just because you are trying to stay in bed too long or at times when you would normally be awake, see your doctor.

Your goal is to learn to associate being in bed with being sleepy, not with the frustration that occurs with difficulty getting to sleep. You must learn to deal with this in a way that will not perpetuate the problem. This means breaking the cycle at least six times out of every 10 nights.

Notes or decisions about getting to sleep
1.
2.
3.

But...?

'I can't do this. I'm tired enough already without getting back up again.'
Hard though it seems, you'll be in an even worse state if this problem persists.

'I've tried this before, and it doesn't work.'
Most people who suffer from insomnia have read about this technique, tried it, and concluded that it doesn't work. However, when further questioned, few of them have done it consistently or for long enough. If you have tried it before and are unable to persist with it, see a sleep specialist.

'I'm too tired to get out of bed and I'm too tired to sleep.'
This is the most common complaint about this technique. This sensation is usually experienced when you are drifting in and out of stage one sleep, but, because of the loss of memory that comes with the onset of sleep, you're unaware of it. There are three solutions, none of which sound very convincing. You can reassure yourself that you're going in and out of sleep, and stay in bed. You can force yourself to get up, knowing that this sensation means you're close to good sleep. Or you can decide that this technique is not for you, and choose another.

Workspace for Night Ten

1. Make a list of the things that you could do if you have to get out of bed in the middle of the night.

2. If it would be helpful, prepare some activity in advance.

In conclusion

One of the problems of insomnia is that it generates bad habits. Today we've covered some of the ways to counteract those bad habits. Used persistently, they'll take away some of the causes of insomnia.

IN THE LAST 24 HOURS	YES	NO
Was your actual time in bed within 20 minutes of your preferred time in bed?	▣	☐
Were you ever inappropriately sleepy?	☐	▣
Was your actual bedtime within 30 minutes of your preferred bedtime?	▣	☐
Did you drink caffeine within 10 hours of bedtime?	☐	▣
Are you a non-smoker, a smoker who did not smoke, or, if you are a smoker, did you increase the average time between cigarettes by more than five minutes?	▣	☐
Did you do any of the activities from Night Five (exercise, something fun, something for yourself, something charitable or for others, something peaceful or spiritual)?	▣	☐
Did you work at night, in the evening, or the early morning and take a nap?	▣	☐
Did you sleep at night and also take a nap during the day?	☐	▣
Were you satisfied with the comfort, light, heat, and noise in your bedroom?	▣	☐
Did you watch television in the 30 minutes before you went to sleep?	☐	▣

Count the number of ticks or crosses in the shaded squares to find your total points for the day. Write your score in the box below, and also in the summary table on page 163 .

Total points for today: ☐

NIGHT ELEVEN: SEE THE LIGHT!

We all have natural biological rhythms that are responsible for co-ordinating some of our physiological processes (hormone production, digestion, and sleep) and some of our behaviour (eating, sleep). For most people, surprising though it might seem, our natural rhythm is slightly longer than 24 hours, and it needs to be reset every day, mostly by exposure to light. Of course, this is not a very precise clock, so we are capable of adjusting by an hour or so without much difficulty. However, shift work tends to put the natural clock and our behaviour out of synch for up to several hours, so that our bodies perform badly and rebel.

In addition, some people (morning types or larks) have an early clock that encourages early awakening, while others (evening types or night owls) have a late clock that is also easily delayed. The latter type prefers to stay up late and sleep in until noon. Much has been made of this distinction but, of course, most people are somewhere between the two, or have only slight tendencies towards one or other type. Some people exhibit characteristics of both; for example, preferring to stay up late but being most productive in the late morning. Just as you'd expect, we're all different, but some of the general principles are helpful, especially to shift-workers.

> Use bright light: *early* for day schedules, and *late* for evening schedules.

Today we'll try to make the most of the relationship between your social rhythm and your **circadian rhythm**, one of your biological rhythms with a cycle lasting about a day. This may mean trying to change your circadian rhythm, or adapting your sleep patterns to the rhythm.

- In an ideal world, with everything fitting in with your schedule, when would you prefer to go to bed and get up? When you are on holiday, what time do you go to bed? At what time of the day are you at your most alert and productive?

- Do what you can to set your natural rhythm appropriately:

- If you are an evening type who needs to get up early, try to obtain outside light in the early morning and avoid outside light in the evening.
- If you are a morning type who wakes up too early in the morning, get your outside exposure in the late afternoon or evening and avoid the great outdoors for the first two hours or so after you first wake up in the morning.
- If you are a night-worker who wants to sleep well in the morning, avoid bright light on the way home from work. Wear dark glasses, providing they don't make you too sleepy or obscure your view.
- For the exposure to bright light to have any effect, it should last at least 30 minutes. Good ways to do this include going for a walk or exercising, eating a meal outside, or sitting next to a sunny window.
- Although outdoor light may appear only slightly brighter than indoor light it is, in fact, many times brighter. Indoor light requires much longer to reset your rhythm, and is effective only when your exposure to brighter light is limited.
- You may be tempted to build your own light-box, but the commercial systems have been designed not only to produce the right intensity of light, but also to eliminate dangerous ultraviolet. frequencies.
- People with depression, other psychiatric disorders, or seizures should be careful about manipulating their exposure to light.

Your goal is to use light wisely and appropriately, at least four days out of every five.

Notes or decisions about using light to reset my natural rhythm

1.

2.

3.

But...?

'I can't avoid bright light in the morning after working all night. I have to drive home.'

This is a problem, but you can avoid unnecessary time in the light by going straight to your car and avoiding chores or diversions on the way home. Some people suggest wearing sunglasses, but it may be more important to avoid sleepiness or poor vision when you are driving home after a night shift.

Workspace for Night Eleven

Quiz

1. I work at night. I should avoid exposure to light in the

2. I work days but my sleep is poor. I should seek exposure to the light in the

3. Which of the following are ways to obtain exposure to light?:

    Going for a walk, even if it is cloudy.

    Sitting close to a window while eating a meal.

    Using an expensive box that provides natural light frequencies without harmful ultraviolet.

    Using special goggles that direct light into my eyes.

    All of the above.

In conclusion

We have now completed the topics about timing and sleep. You may need to readdress your preferred time in bed, your bedtime, and perhaps your use of naps. For the rest of the programme we'll be working on the **quality** of sleep.

IN THE LAST 24 HOURS	YES	NO
Was your actual time in bed within 20 minutes of your preferred time in bed?	▓	☐
Were you ever inappropriately sleepy?	☐	▓
Was your actual bedtime within 30 minutes of your preferred bedtime?	▓	☐
Did you drink caffeine within 10 hours of bedtime?	☐	▓
Are you a non-smoker, a smoker who did not smoke or, if you are a smoker, did you increase the average time between cigarettes by more than five minutes?	▓	☐
Did you do any of the activities from Night Five (exercise, something fun, something for yourself, something charitable or for others, something peaceful or spiritual)?	▓	☐
Did you work at night, in the evening, or the early morning and take a nap?	▓	☐
Did you sleep at night and also take a nap during the day?	☐	▓
Were you satisfied with the comfort, light, heat, and noise in your bedroom?	▓	☐
Did you watch television in the 30 minutes before you went to sleep?	☐	▓
Did you stay in bed for longer than 30 minutes without sleep being imminent?	☐	▓

Count the number of ticks or crosses in the shaded squares to find your total points for the day. Write your score in the box below, and also in the summary table on page 163.

Total points for today: ☐

If you've scored five points or fewer you should go back and repeat some of the work on earlier topics.

NIGHT TWELVE: YOU AND YOUR SLEEPING PARTNER

Sleeping with a partner can be advantageous (more people who sleep alone have sleep problems), but it can also be a liability. We have to adjust to sleeping with someone else, and sometimes our partner's habits can be awful, or just disruptive enough to push a delicate sleep balance over the edge. Perhaps this programme can be the impetus for the kind of frank discussion about habits that might ultimately result in better sleep for both of you.

We wake up about seven times a night if we are sleeping well, with only those awakenings (usually up to three) that last more than about two minutes being remembered. In addition, we are momentarily roused up to 15 times an hour. It doesn't take much of a disturbance to increase these numbers to a level at which the quality of sleep deteriorates, and in many cases a partner may well be a major contributing factor.

> **Find a solution that benefits you both.**

Today we'll deal with some simple solutions that should be acceptable to both of you. We'll also address some more controversial issues which might require **negotiation** (communication to arrive at a settlement or agreement) and, with any luck, a **win–win solution** (one in which both participants feel that the result serves their needs).

- Don't let the search for solutions become part of the problem. Accept that attributing blame or fault is unlikely to be helpful, and that the best solution is likely to be one in which you both obtain some benefit.
- Do you sleep better or worse when you're away from home? Also, do you sleep better or worse when you're sleeping without your partner? Discuss the problem with him or her and determine whether this is a scheduling problem, a problem of sleeping conditions, or a problem with noise or restlessness during sleep.
- If sleep schedules are a problem, try to agree on a mutually acceptable plan. Sometimes this will involve different sleeping

patterns on different days of the week. For example, you might follow one partner's schedule on workdays and the other partner's on days off. Other possibilities are to move times of intimacy to a better time, or to ensure that the one who goes to bed later can get ready for bed without disturbing the sleeper. This may mean getting undressed in the bathroom or another different room.

- If noise is the problem, you could try earplugs or a white-noise machine. Some people find that a fan is the answer. Sometimes both partners sleep better if the disturbed partner is allowed to fall asleep first.

- If your partner's snoring or disrupted breathing is disturbing your sleep follow the action suggestions for snoring on page 207. Decide whether he or she needs to see a doctor (use the guidelines given earlier). Strategies to minimize the effect of a snorer include: going to sleep before your snoring partner, masking the noise with the sound produced by a white-noise machine or fan, and wearing earplugs.

- You might also make sure that he or she does not have bad nasal congestion, is not overly tired, tries Breathe-Right® strips for at least five days, and drinks alcohol only according to the guidelines given below. All of these suggestions may lead to an improvement in the snoring – do try them.

- If your partner's movements, especially repetitive movements of their legs, are disturbing, you could suggest making an appointment with a sleep specialist. There are effective medications for these problems. Further details are given on page 213. If your partner tosses and turns at night and is also sleepy during the day, decide whether they may have a breathing problem at night or, indeed, a sleep disorder of their own.

- We discussed temperature, open windows, etc. in an earlier section (Night Eight, page 99) about the bedroom. Now you should consider these things in the context of your needs and those of your partner.

- Minimize the effect of the disturbance. You could try a larger bed, sleeping in twin beds, or even sleeping in separate rooms. If you're considering this, try it for three or four nights and then think about and discuss the pros and cons.

Your goal is to be happy with your sleeping arrangements, having found a solution that satisfies you both.

Notes or decisions about my partner

1.

2.

3.

But...?

'I have no option, my partner determines the conditions in our bedroom.'
If so, there are several things to consider. If your partner's demands are reasonable – because they are necessary to cope with their poor health, for example – you may simply need to be creative about the few improvements you can make to the situation. For example, if your partner needs heat, warmer bedclothes on their side of the bed might allow you to save a few degrees on yours. If your partner's demands are unreasonable, negotiate. If the negotiations are unsuccessful, you have worse problems than just sleep.

Workspace for Night Twelve

Use this space to record each of the issues you need to negotiate with your partner, and the things that you can do about them.

Issues	Solutions

In conclusion

You may not be able to come to an ideal agreement with your partner, but we hope that you'll have finished today with a better sleeping relationship than you started with.

IN THE LAST 24 HOURS	YES	NO
Was your actual time in bed within 20 minutes of your preferred time in bed?	☑	☐
Were you ever inappropriately sleepy?	☐	☑
Was your actual bedtime within 30 minutes of your preferred bedtime?	☑	☐
Did you drink caffeine within 10 hours of bedtime?	☐	☑
Are you a non-smoker, a smoker who did not smoke or, if you are a smoker, did you increase the average time between cigarettes by more than five minutes?	☑	☐
Did you do any of the activities from Night Five (exercise, something fun, something for yourself, something charitable or for others, something peaceful or spiritual)?	☑	☐
Did you work at night, in the evening, or the early morning and take a nap?	☑	☐
Did you sleep at night and also take a nap during the day?	☐	☑
Were you satisfied with the comfort, light, heat, and noise in your bedroom?	☑	☐
Did you watch television in the 30 minutes before you went to sleep?	☐	☑
Did you stay in bed for longer than 30 minutes without sleep being imminent?	☐	☑
If you are a day or early-morning worker, did you get bright light in the morning (but not the evening)?	☑	☐
If you are a night or evening worker, did you avoid bright light in the morning?	☑	☐

Count the number of ticks or crosses in the shaded squares to find your total points for the day. Write your score in the box below, and also in the summary table on page 163.

Total points for today:

NIGHT THIRTEEN: PETS, CHILDREN, AND THE TELEPHONE

It is amazing how much the sleep of parents is disrupted by their children, by pets and the phone, and this problem is magnified many times for working parents, especially shift-workers. Most people would not be expected to disrupt their sleep to deal with a plumber at 2 a.m., but this sort of thing plagues shift-workers all the time. We expect some sleep disturbance, but often, on reflection, we find that it has become unnecessary and avoidable.

> **Don't accept more than one disturbance a night from anyone other than young children.**

Today we'll work out what's disturbing your sleep, and what you can do about it.

- How many times do you wake up during your main sleep period? Count all awakenings, even if they are only momentary. How many of these are because of children, pets or the phone? How many are truly important?
- If you have pets, don't let them sleep in the bedroom.
- Set rules for the phone, and be strict about who is allowed to call between the time when you start winding down for sleep and the time you intend to wake up again. If you expect business calls, make sure that they are meaningful, i.e., that something happens as a consequence of them. If someone calls just for information, suggest that they wait until you are fully awake. If you are a shift-worker, you might prefer to use an answering machine for the time you are relaxing or asleep.
- Talk about how best to divide parental responsibilities for small children, especially if your children are very young. For some couples this works best 'by the night'; others prefer to have one person deal with the early hours and the other the later hours.
- If you are a shift-worker with children at home, it is essential to set some ground rules, with suitable rewards for good compliance. Make at least four hours of your sleep time absolutely undisturbed, with

no visitors, noise (such as vacuuming or the washing machine), and no one coming into the bedroom. Ideally (from your point of view), this is a good time for the rest of the family to be out of the house. You may find that another room, perhaps a basement or an attic room, is a better place to sleep if it is more remote from the centre of activity. When you finally wake up, try to spend some quality time with those who have been supporting your sleep, especially small children.

- If you are disturbed by noise from outside, do what you can to soundproof your windows. To decide how important that is, you might try sleeping somewhere else where you are not disturbed for a few nights and see what difference it makes.

- If you have a noisy neighbour (or a neighbour with a noisy pet), don't just get frustrated and sleep-deprived. Perhaps you can talk to them, or to other neighbours, to see how much the noise is disturbing them. It is better to seek help, counselling, or citizen's advice rather than suffer night after night.

Your goals are to be disturbed infrequently, and for any disturbances that occur to be acceptable to you.

Notes or decisions about disturbance

1.

2.

3.

But…?

'I can't rely on an answering machine because I'm concerned about my family.'
Perhaps a pager would be helpful.

'I have to keep myself alert at night so I can hear my children.'
If you have a partner, it is easiest to divide responsibilities so that you

know when you are off duty and can relax. Talk to other parents to see if your child is unusually disturbing at night. Perhaps he or she has poor sleep habits (for example, too much or too little time napping) which can be improved.

Workspace for Night Thirteen

What has disturbed your sleep over the last week? What can be done about it?

Disturbances	Solutions

In conclusion

You will need to continue to work on reducing your sleep disturbances as we go through this programme. You may want to return to this section intermittently as your sleep changes.

Tomorrow we'll assess your progress so far, and prepare for the final week of the programme.

IN THE LAST 24 HOURS	YES	NO
Was your actual time in bed within 20 minutes of your preferred time in bed?	■	□
Were you ever inappropriately sleepy?	□	■
Was your actual bedtime within 30 minutes of your preferred bedtime?	■	□
Did you drink caffeine within 10 hours of bedtime?	□	■

IN THE LAST 24 HOURS	YES	NO
Are you a non-smoker, a smoker who did not smoke or, if you are a smoker, did you increase the average time between cigarettes by more than five minutes?	■	□
Did you do any of the activities from Night Five (exercise, something fun, something for yourself, something charitable or for others, something peaceful or spiritual)?	■	□
Did you work at night, in the evening, or the early morning and take a nap?	■	□
Did you sleep at night and also take a nap during the day?	□	■
Were you satisfied with the comfort, light, heat, and noise in your bedroom?	■	□
Did you watch television in the 30 minutes before you went to sleep?	□	■
Did you stay in bed for longer than 30 minutes without sleep being imminent?	□	■
If you are a day or early-morning worker, did you get bright light in the morning (but not the evening)?	■	□
If you are a night or evening worker, did you avoid bright light in the morning?	■	□
Did you and your partner keep to a satisfactory agreement about bedtimes and avoiding disturbing each other during the night?	■	□

Count the number of ticks or crosses in the shaded squares to find your total points for the day. Write your score in the box below, and also in the summary table on page 163.

Total points for today: □

NIGHT FOURTEEN: PROGRESS SO FAR

Two weeks in, and this may well be the hardest time. It is time to review your progress again. **Progress** involves development to a higher, better, or more advanced stage.

You should have gained some insights into what affects your sleep health and, perhaps, have started to experience some benefits, although a few people will still need more time to develop significant changes to their sleep and the way they feel as a result of it. However, are there topics that need extra attention? If so, it is still better to repeat sections than to move on too quickly. There are extra columns on the summary sheet for repeated nights on page 163 if you need them.

How well is the programme going?

You have been monitoring your progress on a daily basis by answering questions about the previous 24 hours, and writing your daily scores on the summary sheet. Now count up your total score for the last six nights. Write this total in the box labelled 'Second week total' on the summary sheet. If you have repeated any sections, count up only your most recent points, and make sure that you have a score for each day and have counted only one score for each day. The maximum possible is 63.

- If you scored more than 33, you're doing well.
- If you scored between 16 and 33, you should look back at any topics that are causing problems.
- If you scored less than 16, you need to review and repeat several earlier sections.

What kind of effect is it having on your sleep health?

We can assess your sleep health by how alert you are during your waking hours, and by how restful your main sleep period is. Remember, it may still be too early to see a large improvement.

Answer the following questions by indicating the number of days or nights in the last six on which the following have occurred. Your answer should be between 0 and 6 for each question.

ON HOW MANY DAYS OR NIGHTS	NUMBER (0-6)
did it take you more than 20 minutes to fall asleep?	
were you awake for more than one hour in your main sleep period?	
did you wake up more than five times in your main sleep period?	
were you dangerously sleepy (see page 91)	
were you sleepier than you would have liked to have been?	
TOTAL	

Write your total score on the summary sheet (page 164) in the 'Sleep health scores' chart in the box marked 'Week Two'. It should be less than that for Week One. This will provide another record of your progress through the programme.

Fine-tuning your preferred time in bed
You may find it helpful to adjust your preferred time in bed. Refer to Night One (page 60) to be reminded how to do this.

Notes or decisions about my progress so far

1.

2.

3.

But…?
'I still think that I have a fundamental sleep disorder. Why should I continue with this programme when that is untreated?'
If you have a sleep disorder, you need to go to a doctor and get it

treated. However, almost everyone with a sleep disorder has other sleep issues – the kinds discussed in this programme – which need to be dealt with before good sleep can be expected.

Workspace for Night Fourteen

Let's keep track of the work so far. Which of the nights have been:

	Night(s)
helpful?	
unnecessary?	
unhelpful?	

In conclusion

In the last two weeks we have covered some of the bigger topics in sleep fitness, but the final week may be the most important. That's because all of these topics require time, second thoughts, and refinement. As you enter the final week, pay even more attention to the topics we've already addressed.

NIGHT FIFTEEN: EXERCISE AND SLEEP

Not long ago, advice about exercise would have focused on the importance of three **aerobic exercise** periods each week (designed to increase oxygen consumption and improve the fitness of the heart and circulation). This is still a good thing to do if you can, as it reduces the risk of stroke and heart attacks, but from the sleep perspective it is probably more important to incorporate activity, any activity, into your daily life. The new philosophy is in two stages:

---

1. **A total of at least 30 minutes of any physical activity each day.**
2. **At least three periods of aerobic exercise each week.**

The physical activity can be anything from walking to gardening, climbing a flight or more of stairs, sports, etc. You should do a **total** of 30 minutes of such activities throughout the day, not just a single half-hour block of exercise. So a 10-minute walk to work, five two-minute strolls to your boss's office on the third floor on a workday, a 10-minute walk home and five minutes of gardening would give 35 minutes of total activity for your day. While such activity does less to improve your aerobic capacity than more intensive exercise sessions, it does protect your heart and circulation, and it structures your day and gives you some physical tiredness, which certainly helps to promote sleep. It may also be an effective way to manage your weight.

Don't engage in any physical activity if you have doubts about your health. For most people it is wise to have a medical check-up before starting a new exercise programme.

Today we'll assess your current activity level and plan the kind of activity that will promote good sleep.

- How much physical activity (gardening, sports, etc.) did you have today?
- Aim to walk at least a little every day.

- Always try to climb stairs rather than using a lift, unless your doctor has said that you should not, or to do so leaves you feeling unwell (in which case, see your doctor).
- Avoid strenuous exercise in the two hours or so before bedtime. Exercise before bedtime increases your body temperature and, rather than improving your sleep, it will tend to keep you awake. The exact period of sensitivity differs between individuals, and changes with circumstances (for example, how hard and how long you work out).
- If you are consistently active for at least 30 minutes each day, try to add or maintain three periods of more strenuous exercise, each lasting at least 20 minutes. It is best if this is something that you like to do.

There are many benefits from this exercise. A physically active lifestyle promotes good sleep, helps to control body weight and excess fat, and makes for a more balanced life.

Your goals are to feel good about your physical condition, and to feel physically tired at least four times a week.

Notes or decisions about exercise

1.

2.

3.

But...?

'I know of so many people who have unused exercise machines at home.'
There are also many people who are healthy, perhaps even still alive, because they took their exercise seriously. In general, it's a good idea to establish a pattern of simple exercise (for example, walking, stretching, or gardening) before investing in expensive machines. And don't forget the swimming-pool. Swimming can be one of the best and safest types of exercise.

'I'm too tired to exercise.'
Studies have shown that loss of sleep doesn't affect our ability to be active but it certainly challenges our motivation. You're probably too tired to raise the enthusiasm to get going. Start slowly and modestly. Try to do an activity with friends or one that involves a commitment (a dance class, for example). Once you overcome the initial barrier, you'll realize that the improvement in how you feel afterwards is worth the effort.

'I have a hard time exercising because of pain.'
This is a problem. The first step is to be determined to do the best that you can about your pain. This might mean being more assertive with your health-care providers, working with physical therapists or massage practitioners, or seeking counselling to help you to accept or cope with the pain. Second, find out what exercise is least difficult for you. Again, swimming can be very good in this regard. At the very least, you may be able to manage some stretching exercises.

Workspace for Night Fifteen

To calculate your level of activity, write down the number of minutes that you've spent doing each of the following in the past 24 hours. Then estimate how many minutes that you spend doing them on a typical day.

Activity	Minutes per day	
	Last 24 hours	Typical day
Stationary activity involving more than just your hands (e.g., gardening)		
Slow walking		
Fast walking		
Strenuous activity		
Running		
Sport		
Climbing stairs		
Other		

In conclusion

One of the best things about physical activity is that it does become more pleasurable with time. It is also one of the main components of a balanced life.

IN THE LAST 24 HOURS	YES	NO
Was your actual time in bed within 20 minutes of your preferred time in bed?	▨	☐
Were you ever inappropriately sleepy?	☐	▨
Was your actual bedtime within 30 minutes of your preferred bedtime?	▨	☐
Did you drink caffeine within 10 hours of bedtime?	☐	▨

IN THE LAST 24 HOURS	YES	NO
Are you a non-smoker, a smoker who did not smoke or, if you are a smoker, did you increase the average time between cigarettes by more than five minutes?	■	□
Did you do any of the activities from Night Five (exercise, something fun, something for yourself, something charitable or for others, something peaceful or spiritual)?	■	□
Did you work at night, in the evening, or the early morning and take a nap?	■	□
Did you sleep at night and also take a nap during the day?	□	■
Were you satisfied with the comfort, light, heat, and noise in your bedroom?	■	□
Did you watch television in the 30 minutes before you went to sleep?	□	■
Did you stay in bed for longer than 30 minutes without sleep being imminent?	□	■
If you are a day or early-morning worker, did you get bright light in the morning (but not the evening)?	■	□
If you are a night or evening worker, did you avoid bright light in the morning?	■	□
Did you and your partner keep a satisfactory agreement about bedtimes and avoiding disturbing each other during the night?	■	□
Were you disturbed twice or more by children or the phone, or did you have a pet sleeping in the bedroom?	□	■

Count the number of ticks or crosses in the shaded squares to find your total points for the day. Write your score in the box below, and also in the summary table on page 164.

Total points for today:

NIGHT SIXTEEN: SLEEPING-PILLS AND ALCOHOL

Sleeping-pills, the popular name for drugs that help you to get to sleep or stay asleep, are not a cure for insomnia, but only mask the difficulty you have in getting to sleep. They may hide the real reason for your problems and so prevent proper treatment. Many cause **rebound insomnia**, where you suffer even worse insomnia than you had before when you stop taking the pills. One famous sleep researcher has even said that sleeping-pills *cause* insomnia. For these reasons, most sleep clinicians argue against the use of sleeping-pills for long-term sleeping problems. But do not suddenly stop using prescribed sleeping-pills. It can be dangerous to abruptly change these medications and it is essential to obtain the advice of your doctor.

Some non-prescription medications that are used for insomnia are not, strictly speaking, sleeping-pills. People commonly use **antihistamines**, drugs which are used to combat hay fever and are well known for making their users feel drowsy. Strangely, they are less effective at promoting a good night's sleep.

Sleeping-pills can, however, have their uses. The newer medications are excellent for short-term problems such as travel and managing grief or extreme stress. A doctor will generally prescribe a specific medication for a specific situation, or to deal with two problems at once (sleep and pain, or sleep and depression, for instance).

Avoid non-prescribed sleeping aids, including alcohol.
Don't change your prescribed medications without seeing your doctor.

Today we'll review the substances that you use to help you to sleep, and make some recommendations for future use.

- Have you ever used sleeping-pills or any other substance for the purpose of getting to sleep or sleeping more soundly? Use the workspace on page 136 to create an inventory.
- Avoid over-the-counter sleeping-pills and medications with sleep-inducing properties such as antihistamines to help you get to sleep.

If you've been using these more often than twice a week, see your doctor. Otherwise, just stop taking them.

- Alcohol releases sleepiness and so even a little alcohol can be dangerous for a sleepy person who is driving late at night. However, don't use alcohol to help you to get to sleep, because it damages the quality of your sleep (although you may be unaware of it). It may even cause you to wake up or stir after an hour or two with signs of arousal such as sweating, a racing heart, and restlessness.

- In general, it is considered healthier to restrict alcohol consumption to no more than two beers (or the equivalent) a day for males, and one beer (or the equivalent) a day for females. Alcohol contains a lot of calories, and while moderate consumption appears to give some protection from some heart and circulatory problems, more than the equivalent of three or four alcoholic beverages a day seems to increase blood pressure for many people.

Your goal is to work, with your doctor's help, towards at least 25 nights a month on which you don't use substances to help you to sleep.

Notes or decisions about pills and alcohol
1.
2.
3.

But...?

'Without sleeping-pills I would have no sleep at all.'

Most people who say this actually have poor sleep even with the aid of the sleeping-pills. They have particular trouble because, in the short term, their sleep is worse without the pill, but it will continue to be bad as long as the root cause of the insomnia is untreated. If you have an emotional or psychological attachment to the pills you use to get to sleep, don't focus on them, but attack your sleep problem directly. Seek help.

'Sleeping-pills are the only things that help me to cope with my pain, discomfort or anxiety.'

There are almost certainly better medications than sleeping-pills for these problems. Review your situation with your doctor.

'You've said that I shouldn't use sleeping-pills, but also that I shouldn't stop using sleeping-pills until I've seen my doctor. What should I do?'

First, recognize that you are in a bind. The sleeping-pills are clearly not completely effective (otherwise you wouldn't be taking part in this programme), yet it is not easy for you to stop using them, and you will find it much harder to get to sleep when you do give them up, even if only for a short while. If you use pills every day, or if they were prescribed, make an appointment to see your doctor. If you use over-the-counter medications on an occasional basis, pick a few days when nothing important is happening to do without them.

Workspace for Night Sixteen

Use the space below to list all the substances you've ever used to help you to sleep, adding the benefits and side-effects that you experienced.

Substance	Benefits	Side-effects

In conclusion

In this session we reviewed sleeping-pills and other substances that may help you to sleep, with the aim of allowing you to understand what the best use of these substances might be, and how you could modify your use of non-prescription substances as soon as possible.

IN THE LAST 24 HOURS	YES	NO
Was your actual time in bed within 20 minutes of your preferred time in bed?	■	□
Were you ever inappropriately sleepy?	□	■
Was your actual bedtime within 30 minutes of your preferred bedtime?	■	□
Did you drink caffeine within 10 hours of bedtime?	□	■
Are you a non-smoker, a smoker who did not smoke or, if you are a smoker, did you increase the average time between cigarettes by more than five minutes?	■	□
Did you do any of the activities from Night Five (exercise, something fun, something for yourself, something charitable or for others, something peaceful or spiritual)?	■	□
Did you work at night, in the evening, or the early morning and take a nap?	■	□
Did you sleep at night and also take a nap during the day?	□	■
Were you satisfied with the comfort, light, heat, and noise in your bedroom?	■	□
Did you watch television in the 30 minutes before you went to sleep?	□	■
Did you stay in bed for longer than 30 minutes without sleep being imminent?	□	■
If you are a day or early-morning worker, did you get bright light in the morning (but not the evening)?	■	□

IN THE LAST 24 HOURS	YES	NO
If you are a night or evening worker, did you avoid bright light in the morning?	■	□
Did you and your partner keep a satisfactory agreement about bedtimes and avoiding disturbing each other during the night?	■	□
Were you disturbed twice or more by children or the phone, or did you have a pet sleeping in the bedroom?	□	■
Were you active for a total of at least 30 minutes during the day?	■	□

Count the number of ticks or crosses in the shaded squares to find your total points for the day. Write your score in the box below, and also in the summary table on page 164.

Total points for today: □

If you scored less than eight points, go back to some of the earlier topics before continuing.

NIGHT SEVENTEEN: ROUTINE MEDICAL PROBLEMS

Many routine medical problems affect healthy sleep, whether through disturbance (as a result of pain or discomfort, perhaps), or more directly. For example, allergies and nasal stuffiness can make snoring and sleep apnoea worse.

You have several choices about the type of health care that you use. **Allopathic medicine** is a system of medicine in which diseases are treated by producing a condition incompatible with the problem to be treated. Conventional medicine tends to use this approach. In **homoeopathic medicine** diseases are treated by drugs that produce symptoms like those being treated. **Complementary** or **alternative medicine** are terms for medical approaches other than the conventional Western approach. These include homoeopathy, naturopathy and acupuncture.

> **A healthy body encourages healthy sleep.**

Today we'll review your overall health and make sure that its contribution towards your sleep is positive rather than detrimental.

- Are you healthy? Have you been following your doctor's advice about ongoing minor (or not-so-minor) medical problems such as allergies, athlete's foot, and heartburn? Do you have nagging problems that you have never tackled?
- Have you had a check-up recently? You should have one roughly every three to five years if you are younger than 40, every other year between 40 and 50, and every year thereafter. Seeing doctors for other medical issues doesn't replace the routine check-up.
- Review all the things that you have been advised to do to keep yourself healthy, and make sure that you are taking the right quantities of your prescribed medications at the right times. If you have any doubts about any medication, see your doctor or pharmacist. Think back to the lifestyle changes, exercises, or home therapy that have been recommended. If you're not following the recommendations, seek help. There may be simple solutions to the barriers that you have experienced.

- If you have major health problems, do not put off seeking the appropriate attention. In particular, perhaps you should consider the problems which you dismiss but which make others worry about you.
- If you have minor problems (such as occasional pain or stuffiness), you could try a non-prescription medication to see if it helps. If it does, you should see your doctor for a longer-term plan. Also, consider whether small changes make a difference and adjust your behaviour accordingly. For example, if driving leads to back pain, experiment with different cushions or supports or stretching to make an improvement.
- Review the things you do to maintain good health and avoid problems, especially your diet and exercise. Concentrate on simple sustainable lifestyle changes, rather than dramatic fad diets or dangerously strenuous exercise. If you think you need a big change, it is probably best to see your doctor first and get the most up-to-date advice that is appropriate for you.

Your goal is to develop a pattern of informed, regular, effective medical care.

Notes or decisions about routine medical problems

1.

2.

3.

But...?

'The pills that the doctor gave me just don't work.'

Did you use them exactly as directed? Or for as long as you were supposed to? Did you tell your doctor that they didn't work, or if there were side-effects that bothered you?

'Going to my doctor is an unrewarding experience.'
Then change your doctor. Perfectly competent doctors can fail to make emotional contact with some of their patients, leading to poor communication and an unrewarding experience. Ask your friends about their doctors. If you call a practice for an appointment ask the receptionist who would best meet your needs (explain that you want a doctor who is unhurried, comprehensive, punctual, to the point, down to earth, empathic, a good listener, authoritative or involving, etc.). And persist until your problems are solved. Your doctor's task is to make and keep you well; your task is to keep going and talking until that happens.

Workspace for Night Seventeen

Make a list of your current medical problems and the status of each. Is the treatment successful? If not, return to see your doctor.

Problem	Status

In conclusion

You can't sleep well if you have unresolved medical problems, so today's work has been important. If it means that you can take care of some other worsening issues it will indeed have been worthwhile.

IN THE LAST 24 HOURS	YES	NO
Was your actual time in bed within 20 minutes of your preferred time in bed?	☑	☐
Were you ever inappropriately sleepy?	☐	☐
Was your actual bedtime within 30 minutes of your preferred bedtime?	☑	☐
Did you drink caffeine within 10 hours of bedtime?	☐	☑
Are you a non-smoker, a smoker who did not smoke or, if you are a smoker, did you increase the average time between cigarettes by more than five minutes?	☑	☐
Did you do any of the activities from Night Five (exercise, something fun, something for yourself, something charitable or for others, something peaceful or spiritual)?	☑	☐
Did you work at night, in the evening, or the early morning and take a nap?	☑	☐
Did you sleep at night and also take a nap during the day?	☐	☑
Were you satisfied with the comfort, light, heat, and noise in your bedroom?	☑	☐
Did you watch television in the 30 minutes before you went to sleep?	☐	☑
Did you stay in bed for longer than 30 minutes without sleep being imminent?	☐	☑
If you are a day or early-morning worker, did you get bright light in the morning (but not the evening)?	☑	☐

IN THE LAST 24 HOURS	YES	NO
If you are a night or evening worker, did you avoid bright light in the morning?	■	□
Did you and your partner keep a satisfactory agreement about bedtimes and avoiding disturbing each other during the night?	■	□
Were you disturbed twice or more by children or the phone, or did you have a pet sleeping in the bedroom?	□	■
Were you active for a total of at least 30 minutes during the day?	■	□
Did you use a sleeping-pill or alcohol to help you to get to sleep?	□	■

Count the number of ticks or crosses in the shaded squares to find your total points for the day. Write your score in the box below, and also in the summary table on page 164.

Total points for today: □

NIGHT EIGHTEEN: WORRY, STRESS, AND DEPRESSION

Over two-thirds of the people who have trouble getting to sleep, or getting back to sleep, complain of a racing, overactive brain, or of worry, stress, or depression. It is not always the case that these issues cause the sleep problem, but they certainly don't help and can impede a successful resolution.

Force the issue: fight these fights before you go to bed. Obviously, if you feel hopeless or suicidal, if you have lost interest or pleasure in things, if you have panic attacks with a sudden overwhelming feeling of dread, a racing heart, or difficulty breathing, you should see your doctor to get proper medical attention. But sometimes sleep problems are the primary symptom of depression, or the only one that is not resolved by an otherwise successful medication. In which case, help is needed for the underlying sleep problem. **Depression** is a depressed mood characterized by sadness, despair, and discouragement. **Anxiety** is an unpleasant emotional response to the anticipation of unreal or imagined danger. A **panic attack** is a sudden attack of anxiety with relatively severe physical or mental symptoms. **Stress** is the sum of the biological reactions to adverse conditions.

> **Deal with worries and anxiety before you get into bed.**

Today we'll outline some strategies for dealing with these emotional issues.

- During the last two weeks, have you felt that your brain was too active when you were in bed? Have you been worrying? On a scale of zero to 10 (with 10 as the highest score), grade the stress level that you feel you are experiencing, and decide whether the stress is caused mainly by work, your home life, or both.
- Remember the advice given earlier: get out of bed if sleep is not imminent. This is particularly important if you are prone to worrying or becoming frustrated. It is easier to keep a sense of proportion if you're out of bed and there's a light on.

- Set aside 15 to 20 minutes in the late afternoon or early evening when you can be by yourself to think about some of these issues. You need to tackle them on your terms, when you're awake, alert, and focused.

- Be honest about the things that concern you, and even try to imagine the worst possible outcomes and the circumstances under which they might arise (if you don't do it in the day, you may only end up doing it in the middle of the night).

- For each problem, try to identify one thing, even something small, that you can do to improve the situation and one that represents a step towards a final solution. For example, if your worries are primarily work-related, you might decide to talk to a co-worker the next day, or address a specific and clear complaint to your boss.

- Remember the actions that you've identified (preferably by writing them down), because you may need to refer to them during the night.

- Focus on how you *have been* in the daytime, not on how you *might be*. What, exactly, is wrong after a poor night's sleep? If there are specific problems (for example, if you have falls, make mistakes, or are unable to resist sleep), see your doctor.

- Plan what you'll do if you wake up too early and can't get back to sleep. You could get up after 15 minutes or so, have a bath, or read, for instance. Don't attempt to go back to sleep unless you're so sleepy that you really feel that sleep is imminent. Sticking with such a plan will make you significantly less frustrated.

- See your doctor if you feel that stress or other mental problems are damaging your overall health or well-being. Pay attention to what others say. You may not be the best judge of your mood.

Your goal is to be free from worry, stress, and depression at least nine nights out of every 10.

Notes or decisions about worry, stress, and depression

1.

2.

3.

But...?

'Of course I'm depressed. I can't sleep.'

Most experts agree that mental issues and sleep issues, while closely interwoven, can also be dealt with separately to ensure that both get adequate attention. So don't worry about what's causing what, just begin the process of obtaining healthy sleep and mind.

'There are no solutions to my problems.'

This is simply not true.

Workspace for Night Eighteen

Make a list of the issues that are bothering you. Write down the smallest thing that you could do to make any of these better.

Issues	Actions

In conclusion

We're not suggesting that these serious issues – depression, stress, and anxiety – can be resolved in a single night. However, there are some simple strategies which you can adopt immediately and which will, to a greater or lesser extent, have a beneficial effect.

IN THE LAST 24 HOURS	YES	NO
Was your actual time in bed within 20 minutes of your preferred time in bed?	☑	☐
Were you ever inappropriately sleepy?	☐	☑
Was your actual bedtime within 30 minutes of your preferred bedtime?	☑	☐
Did you drink caffeine within 10 hours of bedtime?	☐	☑
Are you a non-smoker, a smoker who did not smoke or, if you are a smoker, did you increase the average time between cigarettes by more than five minutes?	☑	☐
Did you do any of the activities from Night Five (exercise, something fun, something for yourself, something charitable or for others, something peaceful or spiritual)?	☑	☐
Did you work at night, in the evening, or the early morning and take a nap?	☑	☐
Did you sleep at night and also take a nap during the day?	☐	☑
Were you satisfied with the comfort, light, heat, and noise in your bedroom?	☑	☐
Did you watch television in the 30 minutes before you went to sleep?	☐	☑
Did you stay in bed for longer than 30 minutes without sleep being imminent?	☐	☑
If you are a day or early-morning worker, did you get bright light in the morning (but not the evening)?	☑	☐
If you are a night or evening worker, did you avoid bright light in the morning?	☑	☐
Did you and your partner keep a satisfactory agreement about bedtimes and avoiding disturbing each other during the night?	☑	☐

IN THE LAST 24 HOURS	YES	NO
Were you disturbed twice or more by children or the phone, or did you have a pet sleeping in the bedroom?	☐	☐
Were you active for a total of at least 30 minutes during the day?	☐	☐
Did you use a sleeping-pill or alcohol to help you to get to sleep?	☐	☐
Did you suffer from any routine medical problem (e.g., allergies)?	☐	☐

Count the number of ticks or crosses in the shaded squares to find your total points for the day. Write your score in the box below, and also in the summary table on page 164.

Total points for today:

NIGHT NINETEEN: AVOIDING STIFFNESS, DISCOMFORT, AND PAIN

For some people **pain**, a sensation of discomfort, distress, or agony, can make the night-time unbearable. Even minor pain or discomfort can interfere with good sleep. One particular type of pain that has often been attributed to poor sleep is **fibromyalgia**, muscle pain that is not usually confined to one spot, but moves between large muscles of the body. You may be using a painkiller or **analgesic** to alleviate your pain.

Minimize, tolerate, then if necessary, mask your pain.

Today we'll describe a strategy for dealing with pain that might otherwise disrupt your sleep. How well does it fit in with what you're doing now?

- Which parts of your body are painful, hurt, or are prone to stiffness? Do you have pains that wake you up at night? What makes these pains worse? Use the workspace on page 151.
- Sometimes, but not often, pain can be eliminated. More usually, chronic pain requires all of the following: **minimizing**, **masking**, and **tolerating**.
- Coping with chronic pain is sometimes like being a cross between a scientist and a detective, with your body as the experiment, villain, and hero rolled into one. Probably the best advice is to keep learning what suits you best and focus on the successes, not the failures.

Minimizing pain
This may include a variety of healthy-living strategies.

- Avoid situations that make the pain worse; for example, the wrong temperature or a poor mattress. The best sleeping surface for you might be a waterbed, a mattress of a particular firmness, foam, a foam mattress overlay, or a reclining armchair. Advice about mattresses is given on page 186.
- Avoid challenges that make the pain worse, such as excessive exertion, standing for too long, overeating, or extremes of temperature.

- Pay attention to your good and bad days or nights. Perhaps a worn shoe, an uncomfortable chair, or bad body positioning when you sit is causing problems.
- Tone your body. This will minimize the sensation of pain, prevent further damage and make special exercises easier.
- Consider doing specific exercises designed to ease and prevent pain such as lower-back pain. Always seek professional advice.

Tolerating pain

All too often it's necessary to learn to tolerate a degree of pain.

- Learn to have a comfortable mental attitude about pain, using the thoughts and behavioural patterns that allow you to do your best. Frequently this means not focusing on your inability to be pain-free, but recognizing instead that discomfort is a universal attribute. Pain does not devalue the essential you, and it is only one of many handicaps of life. Many people have grown stronger from the challenge of living with it, even though chronic pain is not to be wished upon anybody.
- Consider changing the pattern of your sleep. Since an extended time in one position may be most painful, some people prefer to have a long nap during the day and shorten their night's sleep. Sometimes this nap is most successful in a comfortable reclining armchair; indeed, sometimes the whole night's sleep is more restful in one.

Masking pain

This involves the use of:

- heat and cold
- medication (see your doctor)
- complementary therapies; for example, massage

See your doctor if your pain is unresolved with the resources at your disposal.

Your goal is to have sleep that is minimally disrupted by pain on at least nine nights out of 10.

Notes or decisions about pain
1.
2.
3.

But…?

'I've tried everything for my pain, and nothing seems to work.'

You may need to shift your focus from trying to eliminate pain to learning to live with it. Your doctor's surgery should be able to help, perhaps by putting you in touch with a suitable therapy group.

Workspace for Night Nineteen

Make an inventory of the things that cause you pain or discomfort. List the circumstances that make it worse, and what can help.

Pain	
Makes worse	
Makes better	

In conclusion

We hope that, using the approach outlined today, you'll have less painful nights.

IN THE LAST 24 HOURS	YES	NO
Was your actual time in bed within 20 minutes of your preferred time in bed?	▓	☐
Were you ever inappropriately sleepy?	☐	▓
Was your actual bedtime within 30 minutes of your preferred bedtime?	▓	☐
Did you drink caffeine within 10 hours of bedtime?	☐	▓
Are you a non-smoker, a smoker who did not smoke or, if you are a smoker, did you increase the average time between cigarettes by more than five minutes?	▓	☐
Did you do any of the activities from Night Five (exercise, something fun, something for yourself, something charitable or for others, something peaceful or spiritual)?	▓	☐
Did you work at night, in the evening, or the early morning and take a nap?	▓	☐
Did you sleep at night and also take a nap during the day?	☐	▓
Were you satisfied with the comfort, light, heat, and noise in your bedroom?	▓	☐
Did you watch television in the 30 minutes before you went to sleep?	☐	▓
Did you stay in bed for longer than 30 minutes without sleep being imminent?	☐	▓
If you are a day or early-morning worker, did you get bright light in the morning (but not the evening)?	▓	☐
If you are a night or evening worker, did you avoid bright light in the morning?	▓	☐

IN THE LAST 24 HOURS	YES	NO
Did you and your partner keep a satisfactory agreement about bedtimes and avoiding disturbing each other during the night?	▓	☐
Were you disturbed twice or more by children or the phone, or did you have a pet sleeping in the bedroom?	☐	▓
Were you active for a total of at least 30 minutes during the day?	▓	☐
Did you use a sleeping-pill or alcohol to help you to get to sleep?	☐	▓
Did you suffer from any routine medical problem (e.g. allergies)?	☐	▓
Did worry or stress disturb your sleep?	☐	▓

Count the number of ticks or crosses in the shaded squares to find your total points for the day. Write your score in the box below, and also in the summary table on page 164.

Total points for today: ☐

NIGHT TWENTY: EATING THE RIGHT THINGS AT THE RIGHT TIMES

Our pattern of eating is important because our digestive systems are partly controlled by our natural biological rhythms. These natural rhythms allow us to anticipate large meals by providing enzymes before the food arrives to aid digestion. Unfortunately for shift-workers, if meals are not eaten at the right times these digestive substances take out their frustration on an empty stomach, and then the food that is eventually eaten is less effectively digested.

What, and when, we eat also influences heartburn and acid reflux, the curse of many shift-workers, and a disruptive influence on sleep. **Gastro-oesophageal reflux** occurs when acid escapes from the stomach and comes back towards the mouth. On the way it burns the delicate tissues of the oesophagus, causing heartburn. It may stimulate nerves, causing coughing, or reach the entrance to the lungs causing choking. If it reaches the mouth, you may vomit.

Eating also affects sleep through arousal, which counters the natural relaxation to sleep. Eating a large meal within two hours of bedtime can increase your metabolic rate and your body temperature at a time when they should be decreasing. This makes it harder to get to sleep at bedtime. Strangely, it is easier to feel sleepy after eating a meal earlier in the day. This is because your body temperature is already high and the increased effort to digest food causes a move away from metabolism in your muscles, promoting inactivity and sleepiness.

> **Eat regularly, and do not eat meals within two hours of bedtime.**

Do you know how and when you should be eating for better sleep? Today these issues are discussed and plans suggested.

- When do you eat your largest meal on workdays and on your days off? Have you ever suffered from heartburn, indigestion, or reflux of acid into your mouth? Does this ever wake you up at night?
- Eat regularly at the same times each day, especially your largest meals.

- Don't eat meals within two or three hours of bedtime. Try to eat your larger meals earlier in the day, at lunchtime rather than in the evening, for example.
- *What* you eat is also important. Choose healthier foods, and eat more protein earlier in the day, and more carbohydrate later in the day (carbohydrates can provide some of the nutrients that are necessary for good sleep). Eat more digestion-friendly fruits and vegetables, too.
- Avoid the foods that give you heartburn, especially within three hours of bedtime, and meals that are spicy, heavy, fatty, greasy or protein-rich in the evening.
- Being overweight can cause more problems with breathing during sleep, such as snoring and apnoea (pauses in breathing as you sleep). It may also be associated with diabetes and night sweats. Try to control your weight by lifestyle management that includes a good diet and moderate exercise. If you are on a weight-loss diet, and unless your doctor recommends otherwise, restrict your weight loss to one to two pounds per week.
- Look after your heart health with fewer fatty foods and less red meat.
- See your doctor for help if you need specific nutritional advice.
- Drink more water (but not close to bedtime).

Acid reflux

This is the digestive acid that escapes from your stomach back towards your mouth. Whether you gain relief from antacids, or from prescribed medications, you are better off avoiding the long-term problems that come from the corrosive effects of the acid on your oesophagus.

- Reflux is made worse by sleep apnoea: if you snore or have pauses in your breathing at night *and* you are too sleepy during the day, you should see your doctor.
- If reflux is a particular problem when you are in bed, you could try raising the head of your bed by placing four- to six-inch blocks under the legs of the bed. This gentle slope will reduce the rate and severity of reflux. Pillows or wedges are much less effective, and may even make things worse because of the way they bend your body at the waist.

156 THE SLEEP SOLUTION

Your goal is to have primary sleep that is undisturbed by the results of eating or digestion, and a bright wakefulness undimmed by poor eating habits.

Notes or decisions about eating

1.

2.

3.

But...?

'My work schedule dictates when I eat. I have no choice.'

You may have no choice about when you eat, but you can control what you eat. Plan appropriate snacks and meals to eat during breaks in your schedule.

Workspace for Night Twenty

List five improvements you could make which would permanently improve your diet or eating habits.

1.
2.
3.
4.
5.

In conclusion

Now we've covered the main issues involved in the 'Twenty-one nights to a better sleep' programme. Tomorrow we'll do the final assessments, and suggest plans for the future.

IN THE LAST 24 HOURS	YES	NO
Was your actual time in bed within 20 minutes of your preferred time in bed?	☑	☐
Were you ever inappropriately sleepy?	☐	☐
Was your actual bedtime within 30 minutes of your preferred bedtime?	☑	☐
Did you drink caffeine within 10 hours of bedtime?	☐	☐
Are you a non-smoker, a smoker who did not smoke or, if you are a smoker, did you increase the average time between cigarettes by more than five minutes?	☑	☐
Did you do any of the activities from Night Five (exercise, something fun, something for yourself, something charitable or for others, something peaceful or spiritual)?	☑	☐
Did you work at night, in the evening, or the early morning and take a nap?	☑	☐
Did you sleep at night and also take a nap during the day?	☐	☑
Were you satisfied with the comfort, light, heat, and noise in your bedroom?	☑	☐
Did you watch television in the 30 minutes before you went to sleep?	☐	☐
Did you stay in bed for longer than 30 minutes without sleep being imminent?	☐	☑
If you are a day or early-morning worker, did you get bright light in the morning (but not the evening)?	☑	☐

IN THE LAST 24 HOURS	YES	NO
If you are a night or evening worker, did you avoid bright light in the morning?	▓	☐
Did you and your partner keep a satisfactory agreement about bedtimes and avoiding disturbing each other during the night?	▓	☐
Were you disturbed twice or more by children or the phone, or did you have a pet sleeping in the bedroom?	☐	▓
Were you active for a total of at least 30 minutes during the day?	▓	☐
Did you use a sleeping-pill or alcohol to help you to get to sleep?	☐	▓
Did you suffer from any routine medical problem (e.g. allergies)?	☐	▓
Did worry or stress disturb your sleep?	☐	▓
Did pain wake you up during the night?	☐	▓

Count the number of ticks or crosses in the shaded squares to find your total points for the day. Write your score in the box below, and also in the summary table on page 164.

Total points for today: ☐

NIGHT TWENTY-ONE: AN END ... AND A NEW BEGINNING

How well have you done? By now there should have been positive changes to your sleep, and you should have gained some insights into what affects your sleep health.

It's now time for the final evaluations in which your efforts over the last 21 nights will be assessed.

IN THE LAST 24 HOURS	YES	NO
Was your actual time in bed within 20 minutes of your preferred time in bed?	■	□
Were you ever inappropriately sleepy?	□	■
Was your actual bedtime within 30 minutes of your preferred bedtime?	■	□
Did you drink caffeine within 10 hours of bedtime?	□	■
Are you a non-smoker, a smoker who did not smoke or, if you are a smoker, did you increase the average time between cigarettes by more than five minutes?	■	□
Did you do any of the activities from Night Five (exercise, something fun, something for yourself, something charitable or for others, something peaceful or spiritual)?	■	□
Did you work at night, in the evening, or the early morning and take a nap?	■	□
Did you sleep at night and also take a nap during the day?	□	■
Were you satisfied with the comfort, light, heat, and noise in your bedroom?	■	□
Did you watch television in the 30 minutes before you went to sleep?	□	■
Did you stay in bed for longer than 30 minutes without sleep being imminent?	□	■

IN THE LAST 24 HOURS	YES	NO
If you are a day or early-morning worker, did you get bright light in the morning (but not the evening)?	■	□
If you are a night or evening worker, did you avoid bright light in the morning?	■	□
Did you and your partner keep a satisfactory agreement about bedtimes and avoiding disturbing each other during the night?	■	□
Were you disturbed twice or more by children or the phone, or did you have a pet sleeping in the bedroom?	□	■
Were you active for a total of at least 30 minutes during the day?	■	□
Did you use a sleeping-pill or alcohol to help you to get to sleep?	□	■
Did you suffer from any routine medical problem (e.g. allergies)?	□	■
Did worry or stress disturb your sleep?	□	■
Did pain wake you up during the night?	□	■
Did heartburn or reflux interfere with your sleep?	□	■

Count the number of ticks or crosses in the shaded squares to find your total points for the day. Write your score in the box below, and also in the summary table on page 164.

Total points for today: □

How well have you done?

Count up your total points for the last seven days (including today) as listed on the summary sheet. Write this total in the box labelled 'Third week total' on the summary sheet. If you have repeated any sections, count only the most recent points, but make sure that you have a score for each day. The maximum possible score is 119.

- If you scored more than 58, you have done very well.
- If you scored between 30 and 57, you are on track. You've learnt some important lessons, and, with a little persistence, you should continue to improve.
- If you scored less than 29, you need to review and repeat some of the earlier sections.

What effect is the programme having on your sleep health?

We can assess your sleep health by how alert you are during your waking hours, and by how restful your main sleep period is.

Answer the following questions by indicating the number of days or nights in the last six on which the following have occurred. Your answer should be between zero and six for each question.

ON HOW MANY DAYS OR NIGHTS	NUMBER (0-6)
did it take you more than 20 minutes to fall asleep?	
were you awake for more than one hour in your main sleep period?	
did you wake up more than five times in your main sleep period?	
were you dangerously sleepy (see page 91)?	
were you sleepier than you would have liked to have been?	
TOTAL	

Write this total on the summary sheet in the 'Sleep health scores' chart, in the box marked 'Week Three'. If things have gone well, it should be between zero and nine and less than the values for Weeks One and Two.

What you have learned

We hope that you are satisfied with your improved sleep, and with feeling better during the day. Many of you will have achieved only a partial improvement in these three weeks, and will need to persist with the exercises outlined in this programme for a much longer period. Please use Chapter 7: Sleep Tips – to supplement this programme; it provides advice about topics which couldn't be covered here.

PROGRAMME SUMMARY SHEET

Daily points scores

Write your scores from the 'In the last 24 hours' questionnaires in this table. At the end of each week calculate your total score. Use the extra columns – (b), (c) and (d) – if you repeated days or sections. Calculate your totals using one (the most recent) value from each night.

	POINTS	EXTRA COLUMNS		
		(b)	(c)	(d)
Night 2				
Night 3				
Night 4				
Night 5				
Night 6				
FIRST WEEK TOTAL:				

	POINTS	EXTRA COLUMNS		
		(b)	(c)	(d)
Night 8				
Night 9				
Night 10				
Night 11				
Night 12				
Night 13				
SECOND WEEK TOTAL:				

	POINTS	EXTRA COLUMNS		
		(b)	(c)	(d)
Night 15				
Night 16				
Night 17				
Night 18				
Night 19				
Night 20				
Night 21				
THIRD WEEK TOTAL:				

See Nights Seven, Fourteen or Twenty-one (as appropriate) to understand what your scores mean.

Sleep health scores

Enter your Sleep health scores in this table. You calculated these on Nights Seven, Fourteen, and Twenty-one. The extra columns – (b), (c) and (d) may be useful if you repeated nights or sections.

	POINTS	EXTRA COLUMNS		
		(b)	(c)	(d)
Week One (Night 7)				
Week Two (Night 14)				
Week Three (Night 21)				

See Nights Seven, Fourteen or Twenty-one (as appropriate) to understand what your scores mean.

CHAPTER 6

Creative sleep

When you can sleep well and feel alert during the day, the next step is to use your sleep in an even more positive way to anticipate future needs and generate an extra level of daytime performance.

Few people think of sleep as a creative process. Instead, most of us regard sleep rather negatively, as a waste of time, a necessary evil, or, at best, lost hours. We have an image of the creative genius pushing human endurance to the limit by working into the early hours of the morning, long after the rest of us have succumbed to the temptations of bed. We all know people who don't appear to need much sleep, cramming more into every 24 hours than we accomplish in a week.

The reality is very different. Most of the people who pace the floors at night are poor at solving problems during the day. They have defective concentration and memory, and cannot think things through well. Although some remarkable ideas may have come out of the midnight hours, most good intellectual work is the result of healthy sleep and clear thinking.

Dreams have a better reputation for creativity, and we've probably all heard about people solving difficult problems in their sleep. Perhaps it's even happened to you.

To many people the idea that sleep could be creative sounds strange, even funny. After all, who has not tried to explain away some dozing by claiming that they were 'thinking' or 'taking a power nap'? Nevertheless, there is a creative side to sleep: we are capable of doing better at almost everything if we have adequate sleep beforehand.

Preparing for important events

Anxiety about forthcoming important events can prevent good sleep, and these events can be ruined by a bad night's sleep. How should you prepare for special events such as interviews, travel, examinations, and weddings through better sleep so that you tackle them at your freshest and brightest? In Chapter 3 we explained how to avoid problems. The emphasis in this chapter is on how to get more from these experiences than you would even with your normal sleep: brighter performance, clearer memories. We'll explain the importance of preparation, and the benefits that should be anticipated.

The first step is to prepare adequately. It isn't wise to wait until the most important day of your life to begin your work on creative sleep. Like most things it requires practice to get it right, so you should start using it whenever you're going to need to be a little sharper and more alive than usual.

Your total sleep time over the preceding five nights or so will be crucial, especially as these events rarely occur without some stressful preparation or travel. For someone who normally achieves 49 sleep hours a week, three shorter nights can amount to 20 per cent less sleep, which can't usually be recovered in a single night, particularly if that final night is also likely to be bad for sleep.

Conversely, neither is it helpful to have some very long sleep periods within this critical five-day window. You might imagine that a couple of 12-hour sleeps a few days before the event would top up your five-day sleep balance for the difficult nights ahead. But there is a risk that this will destabilize the regularity of your sleep patterns and make it harder to fall asleep on the final couple of nights. Such a strategy may work for you, but it is more likely that it won't. So only use ultra-long sleep periods with caution, and preferably not at all.

This brings us to the regularity of sleep patterns. Normally, as we know, the best sleep can be obtained when the appropriate amount of time is spent in bed and bedtimes are regular (see the first few nights of the 'Twenty-one nights to better sleep' programme). It is no good having late nights for a week and then trying to go to sleep early in order to prepare for an interview! Obviously, we can have some flexibility in our sleep patterns, but, in general, going to bed any more than an hour earlier than the average bedtime of the previous five days is counter-productive.

It may be just as important not to oversleep, especially on the day of the event. Many people find that oversleeping leaves them feeling groggier than they would like. Again, regularity – sticking to the usual sleep pattern – works best.

On the day of the event, or perhaps even on the day before, it can be very important not to be sleepy, and under these circumstances judicious naps may be useful.

Long-distance travel

Sleep is particularly important when travel between time zones is involved and it makes sense to anticipate time-zone changes in the week before. For example, say Jim lives in London and needs to give a talk in Athens at 8 a.m. on a Monday morning. Because Athens is two hours ahead of London, it would be sensible for him to try to ease his bedtime forward over the five days before his talk. So, if he usually goes to bed between 10 p.m. and midnight, he should try to achieve a regular 10 p.m. bedtime rather than working late. If he needs extra time to prepare for his talk, he should get up earlier in the morning rather than staying up late. This will make it easier for him to be asleep before midnight in Athens, and give him a good chance of getting at least six hours' sleep before he has to get up to give the talk.

You can use a similar approach if you're going on holiday. However, if the time difference between your home and your holiday destination is more than three hours you'll need some additional help. First, you could reduce your sleep debt in the 24 hours before you travel. Do what you can to maintain good sleep; for example, don't drink more caffeine or alcohol than usual. More creatively, you might want to start taking naps, even very short ones, at the time at which it will be bedtime at your destination. This is usually more important when preparing for one journey (the outward or return) than the other, so you'll need to practise napping either before you leave for your holiday, or while you're away, but not usually both. Another approach is to begin to manipulate your exposure to light before you travel. Just remind yourself that morning exposure to bright light delays your natural rhythm, while evening exposure advances it. You could, for example, seek out bright light at the time when you plan to get up at your destination.

Power napping

Power napping is an effective and underused tool. Basically, a power nap is a quick, intense nap that dramatically improves alertness. These naps are especially useful for those whose sleep is constrained by a busy schedule; for example, mothers with small children, and travelling business executives. However, the details must be right, and they do require some practice if they're to be used to maximum effect.

Power naps should be short, to prevent grogginess on awakening (which has been called 'sleep inertia'). The exact duration of the nap is a matter of choice, but most people prefer naps lasting between 10 and 25 minutes. Some people believe they can't fall asleep in such a short time, but it's simply a question of practice. At first it is more important to relax and be quiet for a while, than actually to fall asleep. That can come later.

Power napping is not a good idea if you have a hard time awakening at the designated time (it's fine to use an alarm clock), or if you have difficulty sleeping at night after having a power nap in the day. The kind of dozing that accompanies unwelcome sleepiness is not a power nap. That kind of sleep is a desperate attempt to compensate for a poor sleep routine, not a genuine use of creative sleep.

Power naps should be practised and practised. To begin with, try power napping only before relatively unimportant events. As your skills improve, you'll find you can use them to enhance your alertness and performance at times when they are needed most.

Dreams

We all dream. We dream throughout sleep, from the first moments until the last. This is a fairly recent rediscovery. For a long time it was thought that dreams were confined to REM sleep. Before that it was generally believed that we only have dreams in the few minutes before we wake up.

No one completely understands what purpose dreams serve, although it is clear that, when we dream, our brains are active. Dream theorists have put forward all kinds of ideas about their function, from parallel universes to random, meaningless, neural signals. Most people feel happiest with the middle-of-the-road interpretation which accepts that the brain is active and suggests that either our dreams or our memories of our dreams are influenced by aspects of our conscious and subconscious minds. We've all experienced waking up after having a strange dream which seemed to be based partly on our own lives and partly on the last television programme we watched.

There are ways to use your dreams creatively, especially if you treat them as a window to your subconscious. Ask yourself what each dream meant, then question why you answered in the way that you did. See what you can learn from your answers. Here's a simple example.

'I had a dream about an old girlfriend. This is someone that I knew years ago. In the dream we were lovers. I woke up, startled.'

The first step is to comment about the significance: obviously, this description has an element of nostalgia. Why? Perhaps because the dreamer is subconsciously yearning for pleasurable past times. And the lesson? Maybe life is a little humdrum at the moment. He's too focused on routine, and not actively looking for adventure. Maybe he needs to broaden his horizons.

There's nothing mystical about this process. Our dreams have no message. We're just using a product of our minds to think about what's below our conscious façade. There's nothing true or false about dreams, either.

Make a point of writing down your dreams each morning. You'll be surprised at how many more you seem to be having, and how complex they become. Talk to others about their dreams and how they interpret them, and use what you learn to refine your own skills.

Future dawns

You've worked through *The Sleep Solution* and we hope you've developed an appreciation of the benefits of good sleep. We also hope that your own sleep has improved, and will continue to improve as you refine the techniques that we've suggested for sleep fitness.

It is our belief that over the next few years we will see great changes in the way in which good sleep is appreciated and used to beneficial effect. We also believe that poor sleep will be treated more seriously and constructively and not simply shrugged off with a few pills. We hope that *The Sleep Solution* will play a role in broadening knowledge and stimulating debate about sleep. Above all we hope it works for you.

CHAPTER 7

Sleep Tips:
help for specific
sleep problems

This is a self-help section. We have simplified the subject by dividing it into small, almost self-contained topics. Many of the headings are phrases that describe what you experience, rather than the kinds of medical terms that might be of more interest to your doctor. Don't be put off by the large number of topics – it is a complex subject. You can seek out and read only the parts that concern you.

HOW THE TIPS ARE ORGANIZED

The topics are arranged as follows:

To avoid repetition, there is a general list of instructions about when to see your doctor at the start of each section. Only changes or additions to those instructions are given under the individual topics.

For unfamiliar words or abbreviations there is a glossary on page 237, a list of helpful books and articles on page 243, and websites are on page 246.

HOW TO USE THIS CHAPTER

We have designed this part of the book for *browsing*: just dip into it to look for topics that might be relevant to you and your sleep problems.

You will find it most helpful if you think about your own sleep, and how you feel during the daytime, and then talk to others who know you to find out what they have observed. Then start looking up the relevant sections in the book, and try to use the topics to make some improvements. One topic should lead to another, until you really begin to understand what you can do to make things better. Do not hesitate to see your doctor at any time.

The evaluation part of this book (Chapter 4) can also be used to help you to decide where to begin. Any 'Yes' answers should encourage you to look in the appropriate topics of Chapter 7: Sleep Tips. In this section, you may find some statements that appear to be contradictory: napping is good under some circumstances and bad under others, for example. Simply follow the advice that best applies to your circumstances. Remember that the advice is written for adults and does not necessarily apply to children.

Many of the suggestions have not been formally studied under full scientific research conditions. Most are, however, based on clinical experience. Some are deductions drawn from the way we think sleep works. In any case, because people differ in their biological and psychological make-up, generalizations cannot be assumed. Treat the ideas as educational guidelines, and if you are in any doubt about your sleep from a medical or safety perspective, go to your doctor for a thorough medical evaluation.

Our hope is that within these pages you will find the advice and help to let you obtain more satisfying sleep, and that you can awaken each morning for productive, alert and rewarding days.

BELIEFS, MYTHS AND MISCONCEPTIONS ABOUT SLEEP

Some people are more affected by their worry about a sleep problem than the problem itself. Others may not be paying enough attention to their problem, ignoring the legitimate concern of their partners, family or fellow workers.

Goal
A balanced understanding of sleep and its problems.

Action
- What concerns you about your sleep? Use the sleep assessments in this book to check your conclusions.
- Listen to the way you discuss your sleep with others. Do you dismiss their opinions with a few well-used arguments? If so, check that you are not mistaken.
- Focus on the ways that your sleep problems affect your life. A sleep problem is serious if it affects your waking life in a significant way.
- See your doctor if:
  - you think that you have a sleep disorder
  - you have unwelcome sleepiness during the daytime (see pages 46 and 198)
  - you are bothered or preoccupied by your sleep on more than five days a month
  - the suggestions in this book don't appear to make any difference

Preoccupied or bothered by your sleep
You're preoccupied, bothered, distracted, or dissatisfied with one or more aspects of your sleep. These concerns may include poor sleep, unrefreshing sleep, not enough sleep, activity in your sleep, fatigue or sleepiness when you are awake.

Goal
To be concerned about your sleep fewer than five times a month.

Action

- Decide whether you have a *sleep disorder* (requiring attention from a doctor or sleep specialist), or a *sleep problem* (which can be helped by actions that you take yourself). A sleep disorder affects your health; for example, by making an accident more likely (such as from sleepiness or sleep-walking), or by increasing heart problems (through sleep disruption or breathing problems in sleep).
- Worrying about your sleep won't help, unless you do something. Find and follow the most appropriate advice in this book. Even if you think that you have done all that you could have in the past, look again.
- Remember that, although it's possible to see some benefits from the healing process quite quickly, many sleep problems seem to develop and be resolved slowly. Allow enough time for the full cure to take place.
- If you're in doubt, or still concerned, having done everything you could, seek professional help.

I need at least eight hours' sleep each night

You've been told that you need at least eight hours of sleep each night, but you rarely get that much. Should you be concerned?

Goal

To obtain enough sleep to be refreshed and alert when you need to be awake.

Action

- Decide how much sleep you need from the way you feel and perform during the day. If you feel fine, you're probably getting enough sleep. Different people need different amounts of sleep depending on their personality, character and habits.
- Think back to those times when you did feel good during the day (on holiday, perhaps), and remember how much sleep you were getting at the time. What were you doing then that you could repeat now? Or what should you now be avoiding?
- Try slowly to increase the time that you spend asleep to see if it helps (see 'Sleep extension therapy', page 230).

The harder I find it to sleep, the more time I should stay in bed

You might feel that because you have trouble getting to sleep, or returning to sleep, you should spend longer in bed. However, this may prevent you from becoming sleepy enough to get to sleep. It will also stretch what sleep you do get, reducing its quality and making it even easier for you to have a disturbed night.

Goal

To get at least 48 minutes of sleep for every hour you spend in bed.

Action

- To make sure that you're spending the right amount of time in bed, follow the instructions in the first few nights of the 'Twenty-one nights to better sleep' programme.
- If you're currently getting less than 48 minutes' sleep for each hour that you spend in bed, try *reducing* your nightly time in bed by 15 minutes and reassess how you are after a week.
- If you've been in bed for about 20 minutes and sleep is not imminent, get out of bed and do something relaxing until you feel sleepy enough to go to sleep. See 'Sleep restriction therapy', page 231.
- If you're asleep for over 54 minutes for each hour that you're in bed, try increasing your nightly time in bed by 15 minutes. After a week, reassess your sleep. Return to your original pattern if you're now sleeping for less than 48 minutes for each hour in bed. If you're still sleeping for over 54 minutes an hour, increase your nightly time in bed by another 15 minutes. If you don't feel better during the day as a result of doing this, you're almost certainly being affected by another sleep problem.

I don't have a sleep problem – I can fall asleep at any time

Being able to fall asleep easily under almost any circumstances is more often a sign of poor, rather than good, sleep health. Most people who can do this aren't getting enough sleep, or the sleep that they are getting may be of much poorer quality than it seems. However, a few people with reasonable sleep have trained themselves to fall asleep quickly under specific circumstances, for example, on the bus home from work.

Goal

To be asleep in 20 minutes or less at your usual bedtime. There should be other times of the day when it's difficult for you to fall asleep in less than 30 minutes, even if you're relaxed and comfortable.

Action

- Treat the ability to fall asleep at any time of the day as a sign of unwelcome sleepiness. Check out that section of this book (page 198) to see what can be done about it.
- Do what you can to improve your overall sleep health.
- Increase the time that you spend sleeping for a few weeks (see 'Sleep extension therapy', page 230). If that doesn't make you less sleepy, see your doctor.

If I don't get enough sleep, I will die

This myth, believed by some anxious people, has gained spurious credibility from descriptions of an incredibly rare inherited genetic disorder and some extreme experiments on rats.

Goal

To maintain a sense of balance and perspective about your sleeping problems.

Action

- Reassure yourself by remembering the worst that you've ever felt after an awful night's sleep. It was probably not as bad as having a cold.
- The biggest danger is from unwelcome sleepiness (with its potential for causing accidents) when you're awake. If you're sleepy, see a doctor.
- Understand how good your body is at compensating for poor sleep. It will take decades for poor sleep or the effort of compensating for poor sleep to wear you down.

- Even people who suffer from severe insomnia usually manage to get over four hours of sleep a night, although many believe they get less. This is enough to survive and to function, albeit not at the most comfortable level.

My sleep is worse now because I'm getting older

It is a common misconception that sleep must get worse as we get older. Many people in their eighties have perfectly good sleep. However, older people are more likely to have medical problems, and they have weaker and slightly earlier biological rhythms. It's also true that individuals' sleep patterns vary more as they get older.

Goal
To understand that healthy sleep is possible, and is needed, whether you are eight or eighty.

Action
- Make the effort to get refreshing, satisfying sleep at night with alert wakefulness during the day. Follow the most appropriate advice in this book.
- Understand that changes in later life – less time but more responsibility, pain, stiffness, and medications – may be acting against good sleep. Work with your doctor on these other issues, and see if your sleep improves.
- Get 'supernormal' sleep (that is, much longer and better sleep than usual) for a couple of weeks, and see what you learn from this.

BEHAVIOUR THAT AFFECTS SLEEP

You know about healthy eating, and the benefits of exercise. This section covers the healthy and not-so-healthy ways of dealing with the other third of your life, the time you spend asleep. Good behaviour in sleep is a solid foundation for dealing with any kind of sleep problem.

Goal
To have sleep that is refreshing, enjoyable, and flexible. This sleep should produce alert and satisfying wakefulness.

Action
- Keep a balanced life as described on this page.
- Keep regular bedtimes and waking-up times (within 30 minutes). For advice on choosing a sensible bedtime see below.
- Maintain a sensible bedtime routine (page 178).
- If you're a clock-watcher, turn your alarm clock away so that you can't see the face if you wake up during the night. This reduces frustration and shortens the time you'll be awake.
- See your doctor if you have unwelcome sleepiness, or any aspect of your sleep worries you.

An unbalanced life

Just as it's hard to feel good during the day if you have poor sleep, it is difficult to sleep well if your waking hours aren't all they should be. An unbalanced life is the cause of many sleep problems.

Goal

To have a properly balanced life, including – every week – some exercise, some relaxation or fun, a reasonable amount of work, some stimulation away from work, some spiritual or charitable enterprise, some shared experiences (e.g. with your family), and some activity that is purely for your own pleasure.

Action
- Review the detailed advice about this topic on Night Five of the 'Twenty-one nights to better sleep' programme.

Choosing when to go to sleep (regular schedule)

The time when we are best able to go to sleep depends on our natural biological patterns, our habits, the schedule of our waking activities, and how sleepy we are. Good sleep requires a careful choice of bedtime.

Goal

To have a consistent bedtime that allows you enough sleep, so that you always wake up refreshed and ready for the day ahead.

Action

- Review the detailed advice about this topic on Night Three of the 'Twenty-one nights to better sleep' programme. In short, if you have a straightforward schedule:
- Calculate how many hours of sleep you need to awaken refreshed and ready for the day. This may be easiest to work out from holidays or days when you aren't working.
- Settle on the waking-up time that is best suited to your lifestyle and work schedule.
- Work backwards to find out what bedtime is needed to achieve this.
- Stick with your chosen bedtime and waking-up time seven days a week. If you ever have to sleep in to catch up on your sleep, try not to sleep for more than one extra hour.

Bedtime routines

Your bedtime routine comprises everything you do before you go to bed and try to go to sleep. For some people, the routine begins the moment that they get home from work.

Goal

To have a satisfying bedtime, with sleep occurring within about 10 or 20 minutes after you decide to go to sleep.

Action

- Review the detailed advice about this topic on Night Nine of the 'Twenty-one nights to better sleep' programme. Try to establish a regular and relaxing bedtime routine.

Watching television in bed

More and more people have a television in their bedrooms, but this can be disruptive unless you have robust sleep or you use the bedroom television sparingly. The television and our partners' viewing habits can disturb us more than we realize.

Goal

To watch television in bed twice a week or less, and preferably not at all.

Action

- It's best for your sleep if you use the bedroom only for sleep, comfort behaviour (such as dressing), and intimate behaviour.
- Spend some time making your primary television viewing-room (which should not be the bedroom) as comfortable as you can.
- Try not to watch the television in the bedroom for two weeks. This should be long enough to let you appreciate the advantages of viewing television elsewhere.
- If you choose to watch television in the bedroom, limit the times that you use it. A relaxing film at weekends may not be too disruptive.
- If you must watch television before sleep, avoid stimulating or upsetting subjects. The evening news is often especially disturbing.

Caffeine and other stimulants

Caffeine is a stimulant which, while helpful in keeping us awake under some circumstances, may disrupt sleep and contribute towards sleepiness in others. Related stimulants are found in tea and chocolate.

Goals

To be alert even if you don't drink caffeine. To have no difficulty getting to sleep and no night-time awakenings from consuming caffeine.

Action

- Follow the instructions on the use of caffeine as described on Night Four of the 'Twenty-one nights to better sleep' programme.

Alcohol

Alcohol may make you sleepy but, more importantly, it interferes with restorative, refreshing sleep. It can also make other sleep problems worse, and is especially bad for your breathing while you sleep.

Goal

To avoid having your sleep disturbed by the use of alcohol.

Action

- For best sleep, don't drink alcohol within two hours of bedtime.

- Try to have no more than one alcoholic drink (females) or two (males) a day. (There's a difference because men and women metabolize alcohol differently). Avoid binge drinking.
- Alcohol releases sleepiness. Even one drink can make you significantly more sleepy when you're driving.
- Consider joining an alcohol education programme. It will show you the dangers of alcohol, which you can then match against the pleasure you get from drinking. You'll also gain a better understanding of what is an excessive level of consumption for you.
- Contact a support organization (such as Alcoholics Anonymous) if your alcohol use is out of control.

Smoking

Nicotine is a stimulant, which disrupts sleep. However, it isn't effective at combating unwelcome sleepiness. In addition, cigarettes contain chemicals that affect breathing, and so make the breathing problems of sleep worse.

Goal

Don't smoke. At the very least, aim to be smoking less than half of the number of cigarettes you smoke now within six weeks.

Action

- Plan to give up smoking. See your doctor or health-care centre for help.
- If your partner smokes, work on a plan so that you both give up at the same time.
- Never smoke in bed, or when you're excessively sleepy. Don't smoke in the bedroom.
- Think about why you smoke (to reduce anxiety? for social acceptance?), and look for substitutes.
- Don't place too much emphasis on previous failures to quit. Nicotine is addictive, and the right combination of factors needs to be present for you to stop smoking. One of these times you will succeed.
- If you can't stop smoking altogether at present, restrict the circumstances under which you smoke. In order of importance,

this might mean banning smoking in bed, in the house, in the car, and at work.
- Avoid situations that you know will make it very difficult for you not to smoke. These will be different for each smoker, but often include parties and bars.

Marijuana

Marijuana (or cannabis) may relax you when you first use it, but eventually it makes sleep more difficult and can make you over-anxious. About a third of regular users suffer from mild anxiety, depression, or irritability, all of which interfere with sleep. Some users have severe anxiety, panic attacks, paranoia, delusions, or hallucinations. Some regular marijuana users have sustained brain damage.

Goal
Not to use marijuana.

Action
- Give up, or at least cut back.
- Don't use marijuana to help you to get to sleep. Ultimately it will make your problems worse.
- If giving up is difficult, find out about educational or help programmes. Your doctor or local health centre may be able to help.

Mealtimes

Eating affects our ability to sleep, and the timing of our meals and snacks influences the pattern of our lives. Choosing appropriate mealtimes can be important for good sleep, especially if you have an unusual or irregular schedule.

Goal
To eat a main meal within two to three hours of bedtime no more than four times a month.

Action
- Review the detailed advice about this topic on Night Twenty of the 'Twenty-one nights to better sleep' programme.

Too much stress or anxiety

Negative stress is emotionally disturbing, producing more and more physical symptoms the longer it persists. We often deny the stress in our lives or fail to recognize it until it has become serious. It is hard to sleep well if your life is too stressful.

Anxiety is a reaction to what *might be* going to happen. This reaction can be either a mental preoccupation or physical symptoms.

Goal

Not to allow stress to interfere with your sleep more than once a month.

Action

- Do any of the following apply to you?
  - I have physical symptoms in stressful or anxious situations. For example, shortness of breath, sweating, a racing heart, or perhaps a feeling of nausea.
  - Things I do to avoid anxiety interfere with my life. For example, taking the stairs rather than the lift, or avoiding supermarkets.
  - I check and recheck things, such as locks or whether appliances are turned off.
  - I find it hard to wind down.

- Your doctor can help if any of these apply and you think that anxiety might be contributing to your sleep problems or general lack of well-being.
- Rebalance your life (see page 177). It's difficult to address stress if your life is unbalanced.
- Reconsider your bedtime routine (see page 178). Are you allowing enough time, and doing the right things, to wind down after the most stressful periods of your day?
- Consider using some specific techniques for reducing stress, such as hypnosis, massage, polarity therapy, music or relaxation tapes.

If a child has poor sleep

You probably expected that having a young baby in the house would disrupt your sleep. You may be more surprised to find that your sleep continues to be disrupted until the infant is three years or older, and (more indirectly) by the problems that occur throughout childhood and adolescence.

Goals

To have adequate ways of coping with the disruptions caused by young children, and to limit disturbance from older children to a few times a month, when they're sick or especially needy.

Action

- Discuss the problem with your partner and set up a plan or schedule for dealing with your children. If one of you decides to take responsibility for the first awakening, or for weekdays or weekends, the other partner may have better sleep at those times. This will prevent both of you from becoming exhausted.
- Set a regular schedule for your children which allows them to obtain enough sleep. This may mean that they go to bed slightly earlier than they normally fall asleep, but only the regularity of a routine will develop consistent habits.
- Proper bedtime routines for the child are very important. These are obviously age-dependent, but may include putting away toys, then having a drink, a bath and a story.
- Take your child to the doctor if the disturbance takes the form of coughing, wheezing, or complaining of pain, for instance, and you feel that it is caused by an unresolved physical or emotional problem.

You are disturbed by your partner

Most people share their bed or bedroom with a spouse or partner, and this can be a source of disturbance. Incidentally, complaints of disturbed sleep are more common from people who don't have a partner, so his or her irritating habits should be kept in perspective.

Goals

To adopt a short-term solution, and to commit jointly to a mutually desirable outcome.

Action
- Review the detailed advice about this topic on Night Twelve of the 'Twenty-one nights to better sleep' programme.

Worries that keep you awake at night

One of the most common reasons for insomnia is persistent worrying or other mental activity during the night.

Goal

To have your sleep disturbed by worry less than once every two weeks, and for less than 30 minutes if it does occur.

Action
- Move your worrying from the night-time to the daytime by forcing yourself to confront issues while you're awake and alert.
- Make every effort to balance your life (see page 177).
- If one major issue preoccupies you, do your best to resolve it. Use whatever resources are available. There may be an employee assistance scheme where you work, or your church or social groups may have skilled advisors. It may even be the right time to get legal advice or formal counselling.
- If your concerns are more general, or aren't going to be resolved quickly, try the technique recommended for minimizing their effect on sleep described on page 232.
- See your doctor if you feel that stress or other mental problems are significantly affecting your overall health or well-being.

Depression

Moods ranging from simple sadness or melancholy to severe depression can affect sleep. As well as making it difficult to maintain a good mental outlook, they may influence sleep biochemically, because some of the chemical causes of depression also affect the control of sleep.

Goal

To eliminate the possibility that depression is causing early-morning awakenings, disrupted sleep, or fatigue during the day.

Action

- See your doctor if you feel that depression is interfering with your life.
- Lack of sleep may lead to depression or tearfulness. Before assuming that depression is your problem, you need to distinguish between sleepiness and mood problems. You may find it helpful to decide which of the following statements apply to you:

  - I often feel sad, melancholy, or weepy.
  - My mood is worse when I wake up in the morning than when I went to bed.
  - I enjoy life less than I used to.
  - I have thought about ending it all, or giving up.
  - My sex life is worse than it used to be.
  - I used to do things for pleasure, but I just don't find those same things as enjoyable now.
  - I eat or drink to find comfort.
  - My appetite – for food and life in general – is worse than it used to be.
  - I wake up earlier than I would like and I just can't get back to sleep.
  - My sexual drive is worse than it used to be.

It's beyond the scope of this book to determine whether you suffer from serious depression, but if the above statements, even one or two of them, seem to apply to you, we suggest that you see your doctor for a more complete evaluation.

- Combat early-morning awakening by adopting a regular schedule with enough actual sleep so that you aren't excessively sleepy during the day.
- Take a nap if it's helpful, but restrict it to 20 minutes or so and don't become frustrated if you don't get to sleep. Avoid longer naps, because they may interfere with your ability to get a good night's sleep.
- Rebalance your life (see page 177).
- Plan what you'll do if you wake up too early and can't get back to sleep. You could get up after 15 minutes or so, have a bath, read, etc.

Don't attempt to go back to sleep unless you are so sleepy that you really feel sleep is imminent. Sticking with such a plan will make you much less frustrated.

- See your doctor if you feel that stress or other mental problems are damaging your overall health or well-being. Listen to what others say. You may not be the best judge of your mood.

Your partner snores

Snoring is worse for partners who are kept awake or disturbed by it in the middle of the night.

Goal

For each partner to have good sleep, without unnecessary loss of comfort or companionship.

Action

- Encourage your spouse or partner to follow the recommendations for snoring on page 207.
- Try to be asleep before your partner. Go to bed before them, or ask them to stay awake until you're asleep.
- If you have a small bed, consider getting a larger one. It's surprising how much difference even a few inches can make to the degree of disturbance from mild snoring.
- Try using earplugs.
- Maybe you could mask the noise of the snoring with a fan, or a white-noise machine. Audiotapes can also be used if the problem is most severe when you are trying to get to sleep.
- Sleep in a separate room from your partner for at least some nights of the week. You could take turns to sleep elsewhere.
- See your doctor if you can't get rid of unwelcome sleepiness, especially if it does not resolve with a few nights' sleep away from your partner. Take refreshing naps rather than remaining dangerously sleepy.

YOUR SLEEP ENVIRONMENT

Your sleep environment (usually your bedroom) is another important influence on your sleep fitness.

Goal
To have a bedroom that is relaxing, comfortable, and welcoming, the kind of room in which it is easy to feel sleepy and awaken alert and refreshed.

Action
- Review the detailed advice about this topic on Night Eight of the 'Twenty-one nights to better sleep' programme.

Your mattress
Your mattress can certainly make an important contribution to the quality of your sleep. We tend to be more aware of mattress problems when something else is wrong with our sleep.

Goal
To have no sense that your mattress is uncomfortable. You should awaken with stiffness or discomfort only rarely.

Action
- Remember that, despite what many people say, support and comfort in a mattress are much more important than firmness.
- You can get a good idea of how satisfactory your mattress is by comparing the effect of sleeping on another one. When you're away from home (on holiday, for example), or if you sleep in a different room in your own house, is your sleep better or worse?
- Turn your mattress periodically. This can make a big difference.
- If you think your mattress is too firm, or if you are now suffering from pain or discomfort, try putting a dimpled foam overlay on top of your current mattress to see if things improve. These are reasonably cheap, and will help you decide on the best type of mattress for you.
- Futons tend to wear faster than ordinary mattresses. If you've had your futon for more than two or three years, you should probably check that it is still adequate.
- Most mattresses are designed to last about 12 years, but many people keep them for up to 20 years and then pass them on. Is it time you bought a new one?

Sleeping away from home

Most people have more difficulty with sleep when they're away from their own homes and routines. These problems can be minimized by a little planning.

Goal

Your travels should not be spoilt or compromised by poor sleep.

Action

- Think about sleep as you pack for your trip. Take:
  - your own pillow if you think that you will sleep better with it
  - your alarm clock if you are afraid of oversleeping
  - night-clothes that are suitable for the climate and social situation
  - your regular medications

- If you're particularly sensitive to disturbance when you're travelling, take an 'emergency kit' of the following items: earplugs, eye-shades, painkillers, antihistamines, antacids, and an inflatable travelling pillow.
- Think about other changes you make when you are travelling and out of your normal routine that might affect your sleep. Many people drink more caffeine or alcohol when they're away from home, and almost everyone operates on a different schedule.

Sleeping in hotels and motels

What can you do to ensure you get a good night's sleep when you're staying in a hotel or motel?

Goal

Your travels should not be spoilt or compromised by poor sleep.

Action

- Follow the suggestions for sleeping away from home (see above).
- If you are staying in a hotel or motel, request a quiet room. For example, avoid rooms near the lifts, pool or bar.
- Check your room on arrival. Adjust the temperature so that it will be right by bedtime. Ask the receptionist for extra blankets or pillows if you think you may need them.

- If your room is noisy or uncomfortable, ask to be moved to another. Do this during the day or in the early evening, when other rooms are likely to be available.
- See your doctor if you suffer from poor sleep when travelling in spite of following these suggestions.

Sleeping as a guest in someone else's house

To the difficulties of sleeping on the road are added the complications of being in someone else's house.

Goal

Your visit should not be spoilt or compromised by poor sleep.

Action

- Follow the action suggestions for sleeping away from home (see page 188). Pay particular attention to avoiding problems with allergies, if these are a possibility.
- If you are likely to be too cold, take warm night-clothes.
- Get a sense of your hosts' morning routine before you go to bed. This can save the awkwardness of delaying getting up in case you disturb anyone.
- Agree in advance what time you can use the bathroom in the morning and what time you're expected for breakfast.

DIFFICULTY GETTING TO SLEEP OR STAYING ASLEEP

Insomnia (difficulty getting to sleep, or maintaining satisfying sleep) is not what is wrong; it is the result of something, or many things, not being right.

Goal

To get at least 48 minutes of sleep for every hour spent in bed.

Action

- Success often comes from persisting with small changes. Don't expect there to be a single solution for your problems.

- Try to improve the behaviour that affects your sleep. Follow the most relevant tips in the section beginning on page 176.
- Keep to a regular sleep schedule, seven days a week, avoiding the temptation to sleep in for more than an hour or so at weekends.
- Try not to stay awake for longer than 10 or 20 minutes after you go to bed. If sleep isn't imminent, get up and do something relaxing until you begin to feel sleepy.
- Understand the effect that stimulants have on your body, and don't assume that caffeine doesn't affect you. Follow the suggestions for caffeine consumption on page 179. Coffee can affect sleep for up to 10 hours, so, unless it is absolutely essential, avoid all stimulants after noon. (But never discontinue a prescribed medication without consulting your doctor or pharmacist.)
- Are you depressed? Look at the statements on page 185 again. If you think that any of them apply to you, see your family doctor.
- Also see your doctor if:
  - you're too sleepy (rather than just tired)
  - your insomnia is related to obvious events such as travel examinations, weddings or dealing with grief
  - your insomnia is affecting your health or well-being
  - you're preoccupied with your sleep problems

Trouble getting to sleep

You get into bed and sleep will not come, or perhaps you fall asleep for a very short time and then wake up and can't get back to sleep.

Goal
To fall asleep within 10 or 20 minutes of the time that you decide to go to sleep.

Action
- Don't expect a simple solution. In most cases the solution will take several months and involve several different strategies.
- It's important to improve many aspects of your sleep health and slowly to establish a new sleep pattern.
- Follow the general instructions for insomnia (see page 189).

- Don't lie awake feeling frustrated. If you are not asleep after 15 minutes or so, or if you are becoming frustrated, get up and do something that is interesting but not too stimulating. You could read a book, or spend some time on a hobby. Return to bed only when you're ready to fall asleep.

You're sleepy before bedtime, but wide awake as soon as your head hits the pillow

You may inadvertently have trained yourself to be wide awake when your head hits the pillow, even though you were sleepy before you went to bed. The situation worsens as you become increasingly convinced that you'll have difficulty getting to sleep. You may also have found it easier to sleep away from your bed; for example, on the sofa or away from home.

Goal

To fall asleep within 20 minutes or so of the time when you decide to go to sleep.

Action

- You'll need to retrain yourself to fall asleep properly, which will take some time.
- Use the 'Twenty-one nights to better sleep' programme.
- Concentrate on a regular schedule, and spend just slightly less time in bed than the hours of actual sleep that you get now. See 'Sleep restriction therapy' on page 231.
- Follow the advice given for insomnia (page 189).
- Do you experience restlessness, discomfort, or some other sensation (creeping, crawling, or burning, for example) in your legs, which is relieved by movement? If so, you may have restless legs syndrome (see page 214), which can often delay sleep at bedtime.

'Sunday-night' insomnia

Do you have particular trouble sleeping on the night before the first working day of the week? This is part anxiety, part insomnia, and part biological rhythms. Anxiety about work is common, and is exacerbated by weekend sleep schedules that are later and longer.

Goal

To fall asleep within 30 minutes of deciding to go to sleep.

Action

- Maintain the same schedule throughout the week. Avoid going to bed later than usual on Friday and Saturday nights. If you do stay up late on Saturday night, try to get up within an hour or so of your usual time on Sunday morning.
- Reserve some time over the weekend (not late on Sunday evening) for a 'strategy session' where you can anticipate some of your concerns about the forthcoming week.
- Avoid sleeping in at weekends. Sleep no more than one hour extra (and preferably less than 30 minutes) on weekend nights.
- Avoid a 'Sunday-evening letdown'. Plan pleasurable activities or routines. These could include a favourite meal, a hot bath, or a special television programme.

An overactive brain

Does your mind start racing when you'd like to be getting to sleep? This is one of the most common complaints about sleep. Sometimes it's worry, sometimes just 'everything', but always you feel as though you'll never get to sleep.

Goals

To fall asleep in less than 20 minutes after turning your light off. To go back to sleep in less than 10 minutes if you wake up during the night.

Action

- Rebalance your life (see page 177). This sounds trite, but it can have the biggest effect of all.
- One solution to an overactive brain at night lies in what you do in the hours before you go to bed. Organize a good bedtime routine (see Night Nine of the 'Twenty-one nights to better sleep' programme) and follow the instructions for anticipating worry on page 232.
- Don't stay in bed awake and frustrated. If you are not asleep after 15 minutes or so, and you are becoming increasingly awake and frustrated, get up and do something.

- Follow the advice given for insomnia on page 189.

You wake up too early and can't get back to sleep

You wake up at least an hour before you would like, sometimes without feeling sleepy again. You may be excessively sleepy the following day, or simply feel dejected, lacking in concentration and worried about sleeping. This is a particular problem for older people, women in menopause, and those with depression.

Goal

To wake up no more than 20 minutes before you would like, or to return to sleep within five minutes if you do awaken.

Action

- Don't make the situation worse by becoming frustrated. The solution lies in keeping an open mind and making several small changes, not all of which will produce immediate or obvious results.
- Some people get up and start their day instead of becoming frustrated. Others prefer to relax and rest, even if they don't go back to sleep. Try each approach and decide what suits you best.
- Eliminate or mask any disturbances that may be waking you, such as, sunlight in the morning or a dog barking at night.
- Negotiate with your partner if his or her getting-up behaviour is disturbing you.
- Deal with depression if you have it, or if you or those close to you think you may be depressed (see page 184). Seek professional help.
- If you wake up too early only on special days (when you have an examination, when you're going away, or when something important is happening at work, for example), create a special routine for those occasions. It should include completing your preparations for the following day before you get into bed, and perhaps a slightly later bedtime than usual if that is helpful to you.
- Follow the advice given for insomnia on page 189.

You get no sleep, or very little sleep, at night

Sometimes it feels as though you have been awake all night, and if this happens often you'll become both frustrated and concerned about being too sleepy during the day. Either you suffer from severe insomnia, or you do not correctly perceive exactly how much sleep you're getting.

Goal
To do well during the daytime.

Action
- Focus on your waking life, rather than on your sleep. Spend a few days determining exactly how well you're doing during the day. Ask others what they think. Are you sleepy, fatigued, or exhausted? If not, be prepared to acknowledge that you might be getting more sleep than you think.
- Try reprogramming your sleep by improving your waking schedule, and by spending less time in bed (see the first few nights of the 'Twenty-one nights to better sleep' programme).
- Follow the advice given for insomnia on page 189.
- See your doctor if this problem began rather suddenly or after an illness or accident.

THINGS THAT WAKE YOU UP OR DISTURB YOUR SLEEP

Waking up more than once or twice a night means that you may not be getting the consolidated deep sleep that you need to do well during the day. For each time that you're aware of awakening, you may wake up enough to disturb your sleep, without being fully conscious, five to 20 times.

Goal
To be aware of waking up no more than twice a night.

Action
- Try to work out what is disturbing you, and do anything you can to prevent it, even if it's something that seems very obvious.

- Ask your partner whether they have noticed anything, if you are not sure why you are waking up in the night.
- Follow the more specific instructions in the rest of this section and complete or review the 'Twenty-one nights to better sleep' programme.
- See your doctor if:
  ◆ you're too sleepy during the day, or
  ◆ any aspect of your sleep is particularly worrying.

Needing to go to the lavatory more than twice a night

In healthy sleep, under normal circumstances, urination at night (nocturia) occurs once or not at all. There are many reasons for needing to go to the lavatory more often. Frequent nocturia disrupts sleep and may indicate other problems.

Goal

To urinate less than twice during your main sleep period.

Action

- Limit the amount you drink within an hour or two of bedtime.
- If your sleep is disrupted or disturbed, follow the recommendations given in the appropriate sections of this book.
- Do you have obstructive sleep apnoea (see page 209)? Many patients with apnoea have nocturia.
- Some beverages are also diuretics. Avoid alcohol, tea, colas (especially soft drinks), and coffee in the evening.
- If you're taking water pills (diuretic medications) in the afternoon or evening, ask your doctor if your medication schedule can be rearranged.
- See your doctor if:
  ◆ you also need to urinate frequently during the day
  ◆ you're always thirsty
  ◆ this problem began suddenly or is associated with other new symptoms.

Heartburn at night or waking with acid in your mouth

Reflux occurs when acid from the stomach backs up into the oesophagus and even into the throat, mouth, or lungs. It is associated with a burning sensation ('heartburn') or the taste of acid. This is also known as gastro-oesophageal reflux, nocturnal reflux, or GERD.

Goal

To have no reflux at night, or only on the rare occasions when you've needed to eat late.

Action

- Avoid eating large meals within three hours of bedtime. Avoid foods and beverages that particularly stimulate your stomach. These include spicy or greasy foods (Italian, Mexican), coffee, chocolate, and beer.
- Avoid self-prescribed uncoated aspirin and nonsteroidal anti-inflammatory drugs (NSAIDs). However, don't change or discontinue medications without consulting your doctor.
- Try elevating the head of your bed by putting 10-15 cm (4-6 in) blocks under the legs. It takes a few days to get used to the sensation of sleeping on a slope, but most people adjust well. Make sure that your bed is stable!
- It suits some people to sleep on two or three pillows, but for others the bend in the middle of the body restricts the abdominal organs and makes reflux and the breathing problems of sleep worse.
- Get more exercise. Fitter people and those who are closer to an ideal body weight have less reflux.
- If your doctor has prescribed medications to treat reflux, reread the instructions for use and follow them exactly. Some drugs work effectively only if taken every day, regardless of whether or not you are having a problem.
- See your doctor if:
  - you're having trouble swallowing during the day, for example, when you eat or drink
  - if you're coughing a lot
  - if you're using over-the-counter antacids more or less every day or night

Muscle or joint pain at night

Muscle or joint pain can disturb sleep. It may wake you up (so you are aware of it during the night), or just reduce the quality of your sleep (so you wake up feeling that your sleep wasn't as good as it might have been).

Goal

To function well during the daytime with no awakening at night because of pain.

Action

- Go back over Night Nineteen of the 'Twenty-one nights to better sleep' programme, where this topic is dealt with in some detail.

You wake up with a headache during the night or in the morning

Headaches can disturb your sleep and may indicate another medical problem.

Goal

To reduce the likelihood or severity of your headaches by at least half.

Action

- Check your pillows and mattress to see if they're causing problems by forcing you to sleep in an uncomfortable position. The easiest way to do this is to sleep somewhere else for a night or two.
- See your doctor if:
  - the headaches began suddenly
  - your sleep is disrupted by a more or less constant headache which does not seem to improve when you go to sleep
  - you think you may have sleep apnoea (see page 209), high blood pressure, sinus problems or allergies
  - you have problems with your neck or back
  - this problem persists

Dreams that wake you up

Although such dreams can be disturbing, they often shed light on things that are bothering you at a subconscious level.

Goal

To be woken by dreams no more than a few times each month.

Action

- If the dreams are about choking, drowning, being strangled, or suffocating, investigate whether you have sleep apnoea or nocturnal reflux.
- If they are about feelings or emotions, ask yourself whether there's some 'unfinished business' in your waking life.
- If you have a variety of apparently meaningless dreams, consider whether your sleep is being disrupted by something else. Check the rest of this section for clues.

UNWELCOME SLEEPINESS

Unwelcome sleepiness prevents you from being properly awake and alert during your waking hours. It can range from a groggy sensation or unintended head-nodding or eye-closing to actually falling asleep. People with unwelcome sleepiness are at twice the risk of having a serious accident as the average person.

Goal

To maintain alertness throughout the day, every day.

Action

- If your unwelcome sleepiness occurs only when it can be explained (for example, by a particularly short night), make sure that you're doing the right things to be safe on those occasions.
- Ensure that you're getting enough sleep. Clues that this might not be the case are:
  - sleeping in at weekends,
  - feeling significantly less sleepy by the end of your weekend (or by the end of your working week if you 'party hard' at weekends),
  - habitually falling asleep in less than five minutes,
  - feeling much less sleepy when you're on holiday.
- Almost everybody needs more than six hours' sleep, and some

people need more than nine. See page 204 for some advice to help you with this.

- Is the quality of your sleep good enough? Follow the advice in the section about sleep disturbance (page 194).
- Avoid danger to yourself or others. Follow the advice on pages 39 and 200.
- If you nap to combat overwhelming sleepiness, it may be better to restrict your nap to between 20 and 40 minutes. Allow about 10 to 20 minutes after you wake up before you do anything that requires co-ordination or judgement.
- If you are getting more than six hours of sleep at night, your naps are not refreshing, and you are still sleepy when driving, you probably have a sleep disorder.
- See your doctor if:
  - you're in danger because of sleepiness
  - you have unwelcome sleepiness often for no obvious reason
  - you have mild sleepiness that does not disappear with adequate or extra night-time sleep

Narcolepsy

Narcolepsy is a rare, almost life-long sleep disorder characterized by sudden overwhelming sleepiness. People who suffer from narcolepsy often also have occasional short-lasting paralysis on awakening, night-time hallucinations, and a sudden sensation of weakness in emotional situations. Narcolepsy is a specific sleep disorder, so not everyone who suffers from disabling daytime sleepiness has narcolepsy. Narcolepsy can only be confirmed by tests that are conducted at a sleep disorders centre.

Goals

To understand what's happening and obtain good medical attention. To have only minimal disruption of your life. To educate those around so that they are more supportive. To accept and adjust to your limitations.

Action

- Get medical attention. You'll start to feel better once you understand what's happening, and especially when you begin to control this debilitating disorder. In the meantime, take frequent naps and avoid dangerous situations.

- If it's over 10 years since you were told that you had narcolepsy, or you did not undergo tests at a sleep disorders centre, you should get a proper diagnosis. In the past, some people suffering from apnoea or other sleep problems were incorrectly diagnosed as having narcolepsy.
- Become an expert on the behavioural treatment of narcolepsy by the judicious use of short naps (see 'Nap therapy' on page 229).
- **Never** put yourself or others at risk because of sleepiness.
- Also see your doctor if:
  - you were diagnosed without having both daytime and night-time sleep assessments in a good sleep disorders centre.
  - you were diagnosed as having narcolepsy and your medication is no longer effective.

Too sleepy at work

Sleepiness at work does not happen if you have good sleep health. Between 13 and 50 per cent of major accidents are caused by unwelcome sleepiness. Sometimes we understand why we are sleepy, and sometimes sleepiness is a result of choices that we have made. For optimum sleep health, work towards minimizing sleepiness during your working day.

Goal

To have minimal sleepiness at work; that is, no more than once a month and only when you're aware of the reason (for example, staying up too late).

Action

- Examine the choices you make that might be causing too much sleepiness at work, such as staying up too late, or not getting enough sleep.
- Complete or review the 'Twenty-one nights to better sleep' programme.
- Follow the advice given for unwelcome sleepiness on page 198.

Too sleepy when driving

Sleepiness while driving can be extremely dangerous. It begins with a sleepy feeling, but often quickly progresses to head-nodding and eye-closing and a struggle to control the vehicle correctly. One of its most dangerous aspects is the likelihood of 'microsleeps', which are short (five- to 10-second) lapses into sleep. The driver is usually completely unaware that these are happening, apart from having to struggle to remain alert. Up to 50 per cent of major accidents are caused by unwelcome sleepiness. Alcohol, even modest amounts, brings out and intensifies any sleepiness that you might have.

Goals

To be at no extra risk because of sleepiness when you are driving. To have no head-nodding, eye-closing, drifting, near accidents or accidents.

Action

- Think ahead, and play it safe. Recognize and avoid the circumstances that cause you to become too sleepy when you are driving. Take preventative action.
- Follow the action suggestions for unwelcome sleepiness on page 198.
- Make careful preparations before you get into the car. Schedule long trips to make the best use of your most alert time of day. Leave in plenty of time, so you can stop for frequent breaks or even to take a nap. Take what you need to be comfortable and focused (comfortable clothes and shoes, for example) and something to help you through a sleepy spell until you can stop, such as chewing-gum, a drink, or food. Remember that those things cannot resolve unwelcome sleepiness by themselves, however.
- Take a nap before you leave, if it will help. Allow at least 10 minutes between waking up and departing to get over the grogginess many people experience when they wake up.
- Learn what driving habits suit you best for maximum alertness. These may include the following: listening to the radio, music, or talking books; a cool temperature or fresh air; eating, drinking, or chewing gum; talking; stretching, isometric exercises and mental exercises. Some of these lose their effectiveness if done constantly.

Make sure that strategies you adopt to avoid sleepiness don't distract you too much. **Don't use them to mask sleepiness that requires medical attention**.

- If you become dangerously sleepy while driving, stop as soon as it is safe to do so. If you're going to nap, make sure your car doors are locked.
- An unscheduled stop at a motel would be a lot cheaper and more convenient than a crash in which someone is killed or your driver's licence is suspended.

Daytime exhaustion or fatigue

Being fatigued or exhausted is different from being sleepy, although they often go together. If you're just exhausted or fatigued during the day, you won't usually fall asleep if you attempt to take a nap.

Goal

To have no persistent or unexplained instances of exhaustion or fatigue.

Action

- Is it really fatigue, or is it sleepiness? Before you resign yourself to having chronic fatigue syndrome, consider a number of other treatable possibilities.
- If you're also too sleepy (see Chapter 4), the most likely cause of your fatigue is a sleep disorder. This book may help, but if that is not successful, see your doctor.
- Follow the action suggestions for unwelcome sleepiness on page 190.
- See your doctor if:
  - exhaustion or fatigue is associated with shortness of breath
  - immediately, if it is associated with chest pain that lasts for more than a minute or so,
  - if these symptoms are not getting better.

Sleeping through alarms

It is not surprising that people who are too sleepy often do not wake up when their alarm clock goes off. But sometimes others who have few other sleep problems just cannot get out of bed when the alarm sounds.

Goal
To be able to wake up either by yourself or using only a single alarm on at least five days a week.

Action
- Practise good 'alarm habits':
  - ◆ Think carefully about the best time for your alarm to go off. Make this comfortably late, that is, leaving you just enough time to do everything you need to do. You'll have to prepare as much as you can before you go to bed.
  - ◆ Don't go back to sleep after the alarm has gone off. Don't use the 'snooze' function. If you can't stay awake if you stay in bed after the alarm has gone off, get up as soon as you hear the first alarm.
- Work out exactly how much sleep you need to feel refreshed, and ensure that your bedtime allows that amount of sleep. See the first few nights of the 'Twenty-one nights to better sleep' programme.
- Determine whether you suffer from unwelcome sleepiness (see the section beginning on page 198), and take appropriate action.
- If these suggestions don't work, or you need more than one alarm, see your doctor.

Chronic fatigue syndrome
Chronic fatigue syndrome involves persistent fatigue which doesn't improve with bed rest or sleep and is severe enough to have caused a significant (probably at least a 50 per cent) reduction in your average daily activity, including work.

Goal
To be functioning fully again within a few months.

Action
- Arrange to have a medical check-up, and make sure it is thorough enough to exclude other causes of fatigue, such as depression, sleep problems, infectious illness, anaemia, or thyroid problems. Don't expect your problem to go away instantly, even with the right treatment.
- See a specialist. Don't be tempted to push yourself or to try to beat

it with one approach, like exercise, for example.

- The literature on chronic fatigue syndrome is complex and can't always be taken at face value. Many of the articles written about it espouse only one theory and ignore the rest. Become educated about your problem, but be sceptical about any single opinion.
- Follow the action suggestions for unwelcome sleepiness (see page 198).

Not getting enough sleep

You may be excessively sleepy because you cannot get enough sleep. If the problem affects your health or well-being, it's called 'insufficient sleep syndrome'.

Goals
To obtain enough sleep to avoid unwelcome sleepiness and be fully alert when you're awake.

Action
- View sleep positively – it's time well spent if it results in better wakefulness.
- Examine your sleep patterns. If you sleep in at weekends or on holiday and feel much better, you're probably just not getting enough sleep most of the time.
- Streamline your bedtime and pre-bedtime routines to avoid wasting time.
- Plan fairly constant bedtimes, and especially waking-up times, that will give you enough sleep.
- Try to increase your sleep time gradually. Up to 30 minutes a week is good.
- Discuss your schedule with your partner and get their co-operation.
- Follow the action suggestions for unwelcome sleepiness.
- You shouldn't need to see your doctor about this problem, unless:
  - there's a medical reason why you are not getting enough sleep
  - extra sleep doesn't result in an obvious improvement in how sleepy you are during the day
  - you have a sleep disorder which is affecting the quality of your sleep

Unrefreshing sleep

Your sleep is unrefreshing if you never feel as though you have had enough or if you rarely sleep deeply. An unrefreshing night might occur if the deeper stages of sleep are absent because of disturbance, or if the quality of your sleep has been compromised.

Goal

To wake up feeling significantly more refreshed than when you went to bed at least five days a week.

Action

- Particularly if you're too sleepy during the day, you may have one of a number of sleep problems. Make sure that you do not have breathing problems while you sleep or periodic limb movement disorder, for example.
- Minimize the effects of pain and discomfort. Resolve any medical problems.
- Do the things that are known to improve Delta sleep, such as exercise, a pre-bedtime shower or warm bath, a warm drink or carbohydrate snack before bedtime, and having the right temperature in your bedroom.
- Follow the action suggestions for unwelcome sleepiness (page 198) and the behaviour that affects sleep (page 176).

Napping

Napping is any sleep outside your main sleep period, whether scheduled, intentionally taken, or more or less unintentional (for example, dozing in front of the television).

Goal

To need to nap less than three times a month if you are working during the day and sleeping at night. If you are working and sleeping at other times, to nap whenever you feel that it is necessary or helpful, unless doing so disrupts your main sleep period.

Action

- This topic is dealt with in some detail on Night Six of the 'Twenty-one nights to better sleep' programme.

206 THE SLEEP SOLUTION

PROBLEMS WITH YOUR BREATHING DURING SLEEP

Sleep-related breathing problems range from harmless occasional snoring, through partly obstructed breathing to complete obstructions of the airway with distinct pauses in breathing.

Goals

To minimize your breathing problems and ensure that they do not occur every night, or constitute either a threat to your health or a significant social problem.

Action

- Do you have obstructive sleep apnoea? Follow the action suggestions page 209.
- Does your nose contribute to the problem? If you can't breathe through your nose naturally and reliably, follow the action suggestions for difficulty in breathing through your nose on page 208.
- Practise good weight-management (see page 234).
- Avoid alcohol, especially within three hours of bedtime. Alcohol affects the muscles used in breathing.
- See your doctor if:
  - you're too sleepy, or if your sleep is becoming more disturbed,
  - the social consequences of your breathing are becoming unacceptable, even after you have tried the solutions described here and in the section on page 211.
  - you also have heart problems or high blood pressure,
  - you've recently gained weight or noticed swelling (e.g., swollen ankles).

Coughing spells at night

Coughing that disturbs sleep, or is obvious when you wake up during the night, results from an irritation of the airway, often caused by smoking, reflux, or asthma. Coughing can disturb your partner, even if he or she is not aware of it.

Goal

Not to cough at night, except during infrequent episodes of short-term illness.

Action

- Deal with coughing, even if it's mild, because it disturbs sleep and could indicate other problems. Give up smoking, treat asthma and reflux more aggressively, and avoid allergies.
- Don't let pets sleep in your bedroom.
- Coughing or choking can occur after obstructed breathing. Follow the action suggestions for obstructive sleep apnoea on page 209.
- See your doctor if:
  - coughing is regularly disrupting your sleep at night,
  - you're coughing up phlegm that is bloody or foul-smelling.

Snoring

Snoring occurs when parts of the airway vibrate because of a resistance to breathing. The airway includes the oesophagus, pharynx, mouth and nose. As well as being a considerable social problem, snoring can also indicate a serious sleep disorder such as obstructive sleep apnoea.

Many factors can contribute to the development and intensity of snoring. These include obesity, a narrow airway, a partly obstructed nose, a small or receding jaw, less taut body tissue as we get older, reduced muscle tone from alcohol or medicine, and a lower metabolic rate (which also occurs with increasing age).

Goal

To have minimal snoring, in other words, not every night or not loud enough to be a severe social problem or a threat to your health.

Action

- Follow the action suggestions for sleep-related breathing problems on page 206.
- Help your partner to cope with the problem (see page 186).
- Avoid becoming too tired or sleep-deprived. Keep to a regular sleep schedule and take naps if necessary.

- Does snoring occur only when you're sleeping on your back? There are several ways to combat positional snoring. One is to put a tennis ball in a sock and sew it to the back of your pyjamas.

A dry or sore throat or mouth at night

A persistent dry or sore throat or mouth during sleep usually means you're breathing through your mouth as you sleep. This may indicate fairly severe snoring or obstructive sleep apnoea.

Goal

To have no need to get up for a drink or to moisten your mouth during your main sleep period, and no sensation of dryness when you wake up in the morning.

Action

- Follow the action suggestions for problems with breathing in your sleep on page 206.
- Don't drink caffeinated or sweetened drinks. Water is probably best.
- Follow the action suggestions below for difficulty in breathing through your nose at night.
- See your doctor if you're also excessively thirsty during the day.

Difficulty breathing through your nose at night

Breathing problems in your sleep, allergies, infection and trauma (previous damage) are the most common reasons for difficulty in breathing through your nose at night.

Goal

While asleep, to breathe through your nose (not your mouth), naturally and comfortably.

Action

- Consider whether you may have sleep apnoea (see page 209). See your doctor if necessary.
- Reduce the potential for allergies: keep pets out of the bedroom and think about using a hypoallergenic pillow. Some people have benefited from having a small air filter in the bedroom.

- Humidification can help, especially in the winter or if you live in a dry area.
- Don't smoke. If your partner smokes, negotiate a smoking ban in your bedroom, and preferably, throughout the house.
- Try the Breathe-Right ® nasal strips for a few nights to see if your breathing improves.
- Ask your pharmacist whether using a decongestant or allergy medicine for a few days might be helpful.
- Some nasal sprays can ultimately cause more problems than they solve. If you've been using a spray on a regular basis and have come to depend on it, or you still have problems, consult your doctor.
- See your doctor if:
  - one or both nostrils is always or usually blocked (even during the day)
  - your sleep improves dramatically with over-the-counter allergy medications or decongestants (your doctor will work out a more permanent solution)

Waking up snorting, gasping, or choking

This is usually associated with either obstructive sleep apnoea or gastro-oesophageal reflux. For every time that you're aware of doing this, there have probably been three to 10 other times that you were not.

Goal

To have this problem less than once every month.

Action

- Follow the advice for obstructive sleep apnoea below, or gastro-oesophageal reflux (page 196).
- The problem may be associated with a congested or blocked nose. If so, see page 208.

Obstructive sleep apnoea

This is a disorder in which the effort to take a breath also partially or completely closes the upper airway. This may rouse the sleeper, restrict the transfer of oxygen to the blood, or both. It may lead to serious medical problems, can cause unwelcome sleepiness and fatigue during the day, and decreases one's overall quality of life.

Goal
To have no more than rare episodes of apnoea, with no daytime sleepiness or cardiovascular problems.

Action
- If you think you have apnoea, see your doctor. Effective treatments are available and ignoring this problem may put your health at risk.
- The most effective treatment for severe obstructive sleep apnoea is the nightly use of a CPAP (continuous positive airway pressure) device (see page 233).
- To minimize the symptoms, especially until you get proper treatment, follow the general instructions for breathing problems in sleep on page 206.

Waking up feeling short of breath
Do you wake up feeling short of breath? Do you have to sit up or get out of bed to get your breath back? This is known as sleep-related dyspnea.

Goal
To have no sleep-related dyspnea for at least six months.

Action
- See your doctor if the sensation lasts for more than a minute, or if it is accompanied by chest pain.
- Do you feel as though you have a blockage in your airway? Is it in your nose, throat, or chest? If so, decide whether it is a blockage that is present at other times (as, for example, a physical obstruction), or whether it occurs intermittently (for example, an allergic reaction). Try different sleeping positions, air filters, or antihistamines as appropriate. If the problem doesn't resolve, see your doctor.

- Are you wheezing when this occurs? If so, perhaps you have asthma. If you are already on asthma medication, review your treatment with your doctor, especially if you haven't done so within the last year.

Sleeping in a separate room from your partner because of the noise you make at night

Does your partner have trouble spending the whole night in the same bedroom as you because of the noise you make during the night? Do you snore, snort, gasp, wheeze, talk or make subhuman or screaming noises?

Goal

To be able to sleep together with such disturbances occurring less than once a month.

Action

- Follow the action suggestions for snoring on page 207.
- If you're grinding your teeth, see page 219.
- Suggest that your partner uses earplugs, particularly if they are especially sensitive to disturbance. Don't give them the impression that you're suggesting it's their fault for being a light sleeper! Other possibilities for masking the noise include fans or white-noise machines.
- If you're moving around when you make the noise, or if your sleep is not refreshing, see a doctor.

SLEEP-WALKING AND OTHER ACTIVITY IN SLEEP

This section includes the range of unexpected or unwelcome activities (often, major movements) that take place while we're asleep or half-asleep, such as sleep-talking, sleep-walking and acting out dreams. The medical term for these events is parasomnias.

Goal

To have no such events for at least three months.

Action

- Some sudden movements are normal and are not dangerous. See the action suggestions below for sudden starts as you fall asleep.
- Minimize the risk of hurting yourself or others. Move furniture away from the bed, put an obstruction by the door (but not something that would prevent you getting out in case of fire), and sleep alone if necessary.
- Some sleep-walkers respond well to 'clues'; for example, putting a box in front of the bedroom door to warn them not to go outside.
- Avoid extreme exertion, tiredness or sleep deprivation.
- Reduce stress (see page 182). Stress and anxiety may not actually cause parasomnias, but they can certainly make them more likely to occur.
- Remember, someone who is sleep-walking or acting out dreams should not be woken up unless they are in danger. The person who wakes them may be at risk from violence if the sleeper awakes in a state of confusion.
- See your doctor if:
  - you're too sleepy during the day
  - you have hurt yourself or others
  - you have found yourself in a dangerous situation, or have been told that you were in a dangerous situation
  - you have wet the bed as an adult, or bitten your tongue or your mouth while you were asleep

Giving a sudden start as you fall asleep

You're about to fall asleep when suddenly your whole body gives a sudden jerk, and it can seem as though you have been given an electric shock. You may experience flashes of light or brief hallucinations; more often there's a sensation of falling. These experiences are known as sleep starts, hypnic jerks, or hypnagogic jerks.

Goal

To be unconcerned about this sensation.

Action

- Be reassured that sleep starts are not dangerous. The severest injury they are likely to cause is mild bruising.

- Also check out periodic limb movement disorder and restless legs syndrome (see overleaf and page 215).
- Avoid using too much caffeine or other stimulants (see page 179).

Frequent leg-twitching or kicking while you sleep

Do your legs kick or twitch every 30 seconds or so for periods of the night? You would probably have to be told about this (perhaps by your partner, fed up with having bruised shins), because normally you would be asleep and completely unaware that it is happening. This problem is also known as periodic limb movements of sleep, or periodic limb movement disorder.

Goals

To have no fatigue or sleepiness during the day, and to cause minimal disturbance to your partner.

Action

- Cut out caffeine, especially after noon. Follow the action suggestions for caffeine consumption (see page 179).
- Make sure that you don't have breathing problems in your sleep. Follow the action suggestions on page 206.
- Avoid extreme exertion, tiredness, or sleep deprivation.
- Make sure that you're not anaemic. See your doctor if you're in doubt about this.
- Physical activity helps to promote better circulation, which can improve this problem. See the section on exercise (page 235).
- See your doctor if the problem bothers you, and especially if you're taking an antidepressant medication.

Leg or foot cramps at night

These sustained muscle contractions are painful and may interfere with your sleep.

Goal

To have leg or foot cramps that disturb your sleep fewer than three times a month.

214 THE SLEEP SOLUTION

Action

- Drink plenty of water.
- If you are not otherwise healthy, see your doctor.
- If you exercise, improve your stretching and cooling-down routines. Perhaps you are over-exercising? Follow the action suggestions for exercise (page 235).
- Review your diet. Some people find nutritional supplements, sports beverages or certain fruits (for example, bananas) helpful.
- See your doctor if the cramps started suddenly or are persistent and are not associated with exercise.

Restlessness or discomfort in your legs before sleep

This is a feeling of restlessness, itching, discomfort, crawling, etc. that usually occurs in one or both legs when they are motionless. It is eased by wriggling or walking around and is always relieved by falling asleep, but the discomfort may delay or prevent sleep. While it is most usual near bedtime, it can occur at any time of the day. This problem is called restless legs syndrome.

Goal

To have unwelcome sleepiness or difficulty getting to sleep because of this problem fewer than three times a month.

Action

- Avoid caffeine, especially after noon. Follow the action suggestions for caffeine (page 179).
- Different things help different sufferers. You could try warm socks, cool sheets, a shower, massage, or moving around.
- Avoid extreme exertion, tiredness or sleep deprivation.
- See your doctor if:
  - you might be anaemic
  - you have restless legs syndrome and you're using an anti-depressant medication
  - this problem occurs throughout the day and not just at night, and is associated with other symptoms (especially swelling, or extreme thirst)

- the problem is extremely troublesome or does not seem to be getting better

Muscle spasms as you wake up

Muscle spasms that occur when you wake up, in the absence of other symptoms or problems, are most likely to be caused by a trapped or pressured nerve in the spine.

Goal

To have muscle spasms as you wake up fewer than three times a month.

Action

- Make sure that your mattress is comfortable. Follow the advice about mattresses on page 187.
- Increase the strength and flexibility of your muscles. Make sure that your exercise programme is appropriate for your health (seek medical advice if necessary).

Night sweats

Sweating at night may be medically significant if it's so severe that you need to change your clothing or bedding and if it can't be attributed to a warm environment (for example, a waterbed) or to a short-lasting fever. The medical term for night sweats in sleep is hyperhidrosis.

Goal

Not to have night sweats more than three times a month.

Action

- If you have sleep-related breathing problems, follow the advice on page 206.
- Is the problem associated with excessive alcohol consumption, especially close to bedtime? If so, follow the action suggestions about alcohol on page 179.
- To find out whether your sleeping environment is responsible, try sleeping somewhere else for two or three nights, and see if the problem persists.

- See your doctor if:
  - the sweats began suddenly, or you do not feel well
  - they're associated with difficulty in breathing, frequent urination fever, or excessive thirst

Sleep-walking and other actions while asleep

Sleep-walking usually occurs at the transition from the deepest quiet sleep to a lighter stage of sleep or to wakefulness. The walker is still asleep, but can undertake complex manoeuvres. Sleep-walking is known more formally as somnambulism.

Goals

To have no risk of danger to yourself or others, and to have no unwelcome sleepiness.

Action

- Make physical safety your top priority. Follow the advice given on page 211.

Sleep-talking

Sleep-talking is not harmful, but may indicate unusually deep or unusually disrupted sleep. It is also known as somniloquy.

Goal

Not to talk in your sleep or disturb yourself or your partner more than once a week.

Action

- If you have breathing problems while you are asleep, try the action suggestions on page 208.
- Follow the advice given on page 211.

Violence to others while asleep

Violent movements can occur as a result of exaggerated comfort movements (stretching during a partial arousal), thrashing around during sleep apnoea episodes or seizures, because of sleep-walking (particularly if disturbed), or acting out dreams. Don't underestimate the dangers of the violence. At least 13 people have been murdered by their partners while enacting violent dreams. Be especially wary if you or your partner exhibits choking, grasping, or focused blows.

Goal
To ensure that neither you nor other people are at risk.

Action
- Make sure that everyone stays away from the potentially violent sleep-walker or dream enactor. If necessary, sleep in separate rooms until the problem has been resolved.
- Follow the advice given on page 211.
- See your doctor if:
  - the violence seems to stem from acting out dreams
  - the violence is potentially dangerous to yourself or your partner
  - these are incidental actions but they are frequent or more than a mild irritation

Acting out your dreams while asleep

This problem is believed to occur when the brain fails to turn off muscular activity during dream sleep. Normally we are essentially paralysed when we are dreaming.

Goals
To prevent any danger to yourself or others as a result of acting out your dreams, and to be disturbed by this problem less than once every two months.

Action
- See your doctor. Do this soon if you're in danger of hurting yourself or others, or if the problem has begun abruptly or become frequent.
- If you have sleep-related breathing problems, follow the advice on page 206.

Eating while you are asleep or half asleep

Do you wake up in the kitchen, scarcely knowing how you got there? Or perhaps you're awake on your way to the kitchen but are groggy and have no will-power to get back to bed quickly. We do not know what causes this, but there are a few ways to improve the situation.

Goal
To have fewer than one or two of these events each year.

Action
- Reduce stress. Follow the action suggestions on page 182.
- Don't let yourself become excessively tired or sleepy.
- See your doctor if:
  - this has happened more than once or twice
  - you've turned on kitchen appliances
  - you've woken up choking on food or anything else
  - you also have unwelcome sleepiness
  - this problem concerns or bothers you

Wetting the bed
Bed-wetting may have persisted from childhood, but more often it indicates a problem with arousal (your sleep is too deep) or bladder problems. This is one of the more surprising problems that accompany obstructive sleep apnoea. It is also known as nocturnal enuresis.

Goal
To have no episodes of bed-wetting over a six-month period.

Action
- An examination by a doctor is recommended. The various causes of bed-wetting require very different treatments.
- If you have sleep-related breathing problems, follow the advice given on page 206.
- Limit what you drink within two hours of bedtime.

Screaming, grunting, or groaning in your sleep
In most cases, vocalizations in sleep are a harmless (though often annoying) phenomenon. However, these can also be symptoms of a variety of sleep problems including obstructive sleep apnoea, sleep terrors, sleep-walking and different kinds of nocturnal epilepsy.

Goal
To have silent and refreshing sleep.

Action
- If you have sleep-related breathing problems, follow the advice given on page 206.
- See your doctor if:
  - such vocalizations occur more than a couple of times a week
  - large body movements accompany the vocalizations
  - you think that you might have sleep apnoea
  - you have unwelcome sleepiness

Clenching or grinding your teeth as you sleep
Bruxism is a clenching, tapping, or grinding motion of the jaw that can occur in any stage of sleep. Often the biggest sufferer is the sleeper's partner, who is disturbed by the noise, but bruxism can cause tooth damage and disrupt sleep.

Goals
Not to allow your bruxism to disturb you or your partner more than once every two weeks. To prevent continuing damage to your teeth or jaw.

Action
- See your dentist. He or she should be able to recommend a suitable device to minimize the damage.
- Reduce stress (see page 182). Stress and anxiety may not cause bruxism, but they can certainly increase the incidence of it.
- Restrict alcohol use. Follow the action suggestions on page 179.

You wake up confused or doing inappropriate things
This happens when there is an abrupt partial awakening from deep sleep (quiet sleep stages three or four). The main circumstances under which it occurs are forced awakenings at the time of deepest quiet sleep, and extreme sleep deprivation. The problem is also known as sleep drunkenness.

Goal
To have no sleep drunkenness.

Action
- Get enough sleep!
- If you are likely to be woken while sleeping deeply (for example, by a crying baby) and will need to get out of bed, prepare your surroundings for safety.
- Avoid non-prescription medications that might contribute to deep sleep or grogginess.
- See your doctor if:
  - this is a persistent problem
  - you're taking medications (such as sleeping-pills) which might be responsible

Panic attacks

Panic attacks are usually caused by a sudden sensation of fear, dread, or terror. When they happen during sleep, the person may wake up, cross a room, and even enter the next room before he or she is even aware of being awake. There may be physical symptoms including profuse sweating, a racing or pounding heart, tightness of the chest, and light-headedness.

Goal
To have panic attacks less than once every six months.

Action
- Do you have breathing problems in your sleep? Follow the advice given on page 206.
- Reduce stress (see page 182).
- If these events are panic attacks, you should be somewhat reassured. Although unpleasant, they are not usually dangerous.
- See your doctor if:
  - panic attacks continue to worry you
  - you're concerned that you might hurt yourself when you get out of bed
  - they started when you began a new medication, or increased the dose of a medication you were already taking.

Nightmares

True nightmares are frightening dreams with a story-like quality. They are most troubling, and most often remembered, if associated with an abrupt awakening.

Goal

To have less than one nightmare every six months.

Action

- Assess your sleep to decide whether you have any sleep problems, especially those that affect REM sleep; for example, obstructive sleep apnoea.
- Consider carefully your waking life. Do you have any significant psychological baggage, fears and anxieties, resentment and anger, or poor self-esteem? Follow the action suggestions for rebalancing your life on page 170, and those for dealing with stress and anxiety on page 175.
- See your doctor if:
  - your nightmares are severe or frequent
  - they started very abruptly
  - they affect your daytime behaviour

Night terrors

Night terrors are a terrifying 'half-awakening' that have more impact on the observer than on the sleeper. The sufferer may sit up or leap from the bed screaming or apparently in great terror, but rarely will he or she have any memory of the event whatsoever.

Goal

To have quiet and restful sleep with few arousals and no vocalizations.

Action

- In general, the only risk to the affected person is that of being injured during the night-terror episode. Therefore it is prudent to keep sharp or hard objects away from the bed. In extreme cases they may be in danger of jumping out of a window or running into the street. Modest barriers that do not interfere with fire safety should be used.

- It may be possible to extend the time you spend sleeping each night. This will eventually reduce the intensity of your Delta sleep, which is when most night terrors occur. Similarly, a nap in the late afternoon might help.
- Some people have found it effective to set an alarm clock to go off about 50 minutes after they fall sleep. You'll awaken in an extremely groggy condition, but if you can wake up fully, you should be able to return to sleep and have less intense Delta sleep, again making night terrors less likely.

Hallucinations at night

Sometimes people who are between wakefulness and sleep hear, feel, or see things that are not real. In themselves, these hallucinations (including sleep-onset or hypnagogic hallucinations) do not indicate any disorder, but are interpreted in the light of any other problems the person may have.

Goal

Either to reduce the incidence of these hallucinations, or at least to be reassured that you are not going crazy.

Action

- An occasional hallucination is usually nothing to worry about. If you are concerned about them, or if they're associated with unwelcome sleepiness, see your doctor.
- The most likely explanation for the hallucinations is that you have a sleep problem. Your doctor or sleep specialist should reassure you that you aren't going crazy.
- Try to get enough sleep, preferably in a regular and uninterrupted sleep period.

Waking up paralysed (your brain is awake but you can't move your body)

This phenomenon usually lasts from a few seconds to a few minutes, and, although it is frightening, you're in no danger. Almost all of us will experience this at least once in our lives. It is also known as sleep paralysis.

Goal

Reassurance and acceptance, with little or no fear when the problem occurs.

Action

- Usually no action need be taken. Be reassured that sleep paralysis is not harmful and doesn't last long. This should make it less stressful and frightening.
- Ensure that you are getting enough sleep.
- If sleep paralysis occurs more than twice a year, and especially if it has happened as you've been falling asleep or if you have problems with unwelcome sleepiness, you should be evaluated by a sleep disorders specialist.

UNUSUAL SCHEDULES AND SHIFT WORK

Unusual, variable or disrupted schedules, including shift work and the kinds of disruption that arise from looking after small children, put a real strain on good sleep. For this reason, it is all the more important to strive for good sleep fitness.

Goal

To establish a sustainable sleep schedule that does not result in poor health or unwelcome sleepiness.

Action

- Follow the advice in the first few nights of the 'Twenty-one nights to better sleep' programme.
- Carefully choose your bedtime(s), and make sure that you use naps appropriately.
- Avoid unwelcome sleepiness.
- See your doctor if:
  - you can't avoid unwelcome sleepiness
  - you can't adjust to your schedule

Your natural schedule is too late for your social schedule

Do you always want to go to bed *and* wake up later than you should? This is known as delayed sleep phase syndrome, and it can be devastating for those with a rigid work or school schedule.

Goal

Either to adjust your schedule to a more socially acceptable pattern, or to learn how to live with your delayed sleep phase.

Action

- Try to set up and stick to a suitable schedule, with as constant a routine as you can manage.
- Manipulate daylight to your advantage as far as possible (see page 225).
- Do not consume caffeine for 10 hours before bedtime, even if you do not think it has any effect on you (see page 179).
- See your doctor if you have unwelcome sleepiness, or this problem is causing social difficulty.
- If these measures are not successful, seek help, preferably from a qualified sleep specialist.

Your natural schedule is too early for your social schedule

Do you always want to go to bed and wake up earlier than you should? This is known as advanced sleep phase syndrome, and it can have a devastating effect in households where other people have more usual schedules.

Goal

Either to adjust your schedule to a more socially acceptable pattern, or learn how to live with advanced sleep phase syndrome.

Action

- Try to get on the right schedule and stay there, with as constant a routine as you can manage.

- Manipulate daylight to your advantage. Spend as much time as you can – preferably an hour or two – in bright outdoor light in the late afternoon or evening. If you can't be outside, try to sit close to a large window in a sunny location. Avoid bright light in the early morning if you can.
- Eliminate or mask any disturbances that may be waking you; for example, sunlight or a dog barking.
- Negotiate with your partner if his or her getting-up behaviour is disturbing you.
- Deal with depression if you suffer from it (see page 184).
- See your doctor if:
  - this problem is causing social difficulty
  - you, or others who are close to you, wonder whether you might be depressed
  - the measures outlined above aren't successful

Sleep and your responsibilities at work

Most companies expect you to be ready for work at the beginning of your shift, which means being awake enough to get through the work time without being too sleepy. Your company may also have policies dictating what you should do if you become too sleepy to function properly during your shift.

Goal

To avoid any difficulty with sleepiness at work, both from the safety and work-performance perspectives.

Action

- Before you start shift work, find out what the company policy is about becoming too sleepy to do your job properly in the middle of a shift. This information may be readily available; otherwise ask a 'neutral' person such as a union or personnel/human resources representative.
- It is your responsibility to be ready for work at the beginning of a shift, so you should be rested enough to remain fully awake during the whole shift.
- Your company's policy should detail the circumstances under

which you must stop work when you're too sleepy (if others are at risk, for example), and whether you may return to work later during that shift.
- You may also have a responsibility to take action if you become aware that a co-worker is dangerously sleepy; make enquiries about this.

Choosing when to sleep (irregular schedules, shift work)

The times when we are best able to go to sleep depends on our natural biological patterns, our habits, the schedule of our waking activities, and how sleepy we are. Good sleep requires a careful choice of bedtime. This is particularly important, and especially difficult, with unusual or irregular work hours.

Goal
To have a consistent sleep pattern supplemented with additional naps that leaves you well rested.

Action
- Review the detailed advice about this topic on Night Three of the 'Twenty-one nights to better sleep' programme.

When to eat and drink if you are a shift worker

Eating affects our ability to sleep, and thus the pattern of our lives. Choosing appropriate mealtimes can be an important component of good sleep health, especially if you do not work regular daytime hours. This is particularly important (and difficult) with unusual or irregular work hours.

Goals
To be alert under any schedule without the use of stimulants, and to have sleep that is not disrupted by food or drink.

Action
- Review the detailed advice about this topic on Night Twenty of the 'Twenty-one nights to better sleep' programme.

- As with sleep, set preferred time zones for your main meals. For example, a breakfast time zone and a lunch time zone. You can change what you eat in those zones to fit your work schedule.
- Avoid eating large meals within two hours of any bedtime.
- Learn what foods most affect your sleep and avoid them when your sleep is under pressure.

Staying awake at work

Sleepiness at work is never a feature of good sleep health. Sometimes we understand why we're sleepy, and sometimes sleepiness is a result of choices that we have made. For optimum sleep health, work towards minimal sleepiness during the day. It's essential that you understand what to do if you become too sleepy to function safely or effectively at work.

Goal

To have no dangerous sleepiness in the workplace or on the way to or from work.

Action

- Avoid dangerous situations. If they occur more than rarely because of sleepiness, see your doctor.
- Practise good behaviour for sleep, and, above all, obtain enough sleep.
- Learn what you can do to avoid danger. This will vary according to the rules and circumstances of your job, but might include stopping and napping, taking a break, or making your work less monotonous.
- Boredom and monotony uncover any sleepiness that you might have, but what makes the working environment more interesting for one person makes it duller for another. For instance, some people are kept interested by music, others prefer talk radio, while for others any radio is sleep-inducing.
- As you work on improving your alertness, be careful not to replace it with dangerous distractions or irritations.
- Use stimulants (such as coffee), or stimulating activities (such as eating) sparingly and wisely. If eating keeps you alert and focused, choose foods or snacks that don't create other health or weight problems.

TREATMENTS, THERAPIES AND REMEDIES

There are many different treatments, therapies and remedies for sleep, and we can't possibly cover them all in a book like this. We've chosen a few to give you some idea of the kinds of approaches that are being used.

Goal
An informed and successful use of treatments or therapies for sleep problems.

Action
- With any treatment, make sure that you understand what it is supposed to do, the risks associated with it, the conditions under which you can stop using it, and the risks of stopping.
- Make sure that you tell your doctor about any treatment that you are using, even if it is an alternative or complementary approach.
- See your doctor if your treatment isn't working or is making you worse.

Sleeping-pills (and other drugs that make you feel sleepy)
These are medications that have been designed to help you to get to sleep, or which have another main purpose but also help you to sleep. The best use of sleeping-pills is to deal with short-term problems (grief, for example). They should be used for no more than 10 days, and only rarely (no more than twice a month).

Goal
To make the changes that will allow your doctor to recommend reducing or discontinuing your medication.

Action
- **Never discontinue your prescribed medication, or change the dose, without talking to your doctor about it**. It can be dangerous to do so.
- Be cautious about substances sold in health-food shops as aids to sleep, even if the primary ingredient sounds like a plausible

alternative to pharmaceuticals. There is sometimes little control over the purity or labelling of such products, and they may be even less healthy (and more dangerous) than conventional sleeping-pills.

- Follow the advice given for insomnia on page 189.
- See your doctor:
  - ◆ before trying any sleeping-pills
  - ◆ before changing the dose or discontinuing any sleeping-pills you're already taking
  - ◆ if you're sleepy or unable to function adequately during the day
  - ◆ if your condition has not been improved by this book
  - ◆ if you have insomnia which occurs before specific events (such as travel, or demanding days at work), or as a result of specific circumstances (such as bereavement)

Melatonin

Melatonin is currently popular in some countries as a means of changing circadian rhythms, and for dealing with insomnia. Some people hail it as the latest wonder drug.

Goal

To rely more on behavioural change and good sleep health than on any substance.

Action

- Use melatonin only if you're sure that you don't have a treatable sleep disorder, if the use of bright light is impractical or unsuccessful, and if you're certain about the origin and purity of the product. Find out whether it causes any side-effects.
- Follow the insomnia action suggestions on page 189.
- Read the section on sleeping-pills (page 228).

Nap therapy

Nap therapy, a system of using short naps to combat unwelcome sleepiness, can be used instead of medication for some sleep disorders.

Goal

Safe, efficient napping to control unwelcome daytime sleepiness.

Action

- If your problem is unwelcome sleepiness, keep your naps short. Fifteen to 30 minutes' sleep will probably be most effective. You should wake up feeling refreshed and alert, and certainly feeling better than before you went to sleep.
- Allow enough time to wake up fully after your nap before you do anything that requires your focused attention or concentration.
- You could organize your surroundings to help with the nap therapy. Keep a large pillow and blanket in your car, for instance. Is there a place where you could lie down to sleep at work, before you commute home, for example? Perhaps a reclining armchair would be a good investment at home.
- See your doctor if:
  - you still have unwelcome sleepiness, even using nap therapy
  - you're relying on nap therapy and your sleep has not been properly evaluated by a sleep specialist

Sleep extension therapy

Many people today do not give themselves enough time to get the sleep that they need, so they become chronically sleep-deprived. Sleep extension therapy is a planned technique for spending the right length of time in bed without simply 'diluting' the quality of sleep obtained.

Goal

To have enough sleep to function well when you are awake, probably between 48 and 55 minutes of sleep for every hour that you are in bed.

Action

- There are at least two ways of accomplishing this. One way is to start with 'more than enough' sleep for three or four days. This will quickly show you what it feels like to have sufficient sleep. You can then begin gradually to reduce your sleep time until you meet the goal stated above.
- A second approach involves gradually increasing your sleep time.
- See your doctor if no amount of sleep appears satisfactorily to reduce your unwanted sleepiness.

Sleep restriction therapy

Many people with insomnia (or similar complaints) have had the quality of their sleep 'diluted' to such a degree that extra time in bed does not appear to help. Sleep restriction therapy is a way of 're-concentrating' sleep. It makes going to sleep easier because it breaks the link between lying in bed and sleeplessness.

Goal

To have enough sleep to function well when you are awake, probably between 48 and 55 minutes of sleep for every hour that you are in bed.

Action

- Set aside three or four days when you have nothing important going on in the daytime. At night, get out of bed if you are awake and have been trying to get to sleep for 15 minutes or so, and sleep is not imminent. Stay up until you feel sleepy enough to go to sleep, then go back to bed. Repeat the process if necessary. Sooner or later you'll be sleepy enough to drop right off.
- There are two schools of thought about what you should do while you're out of bed. Both work. The first suggests that you should do something that is relaxing, calming, slightly boring, and not likely to encourage you to stay awake. So watching an old movie that doesn't really interest you might be acceptable, whereas watching an interesting late-night talk show would not. Quiet reading is pretty safe for most people. The second suggests that the more active, distracting and unpleasant the activity, the better. So maybe you could wash the kitchen floor, or clean the bathroom (but *not* if you're in poor health – check with a doctor first).
- Ideally, you should undertake this treatment under the guidance of a sleep specialist. Most people find it hard to persevere without some help and encouragement.

Relaxation techniques

These are techniques that promote relaxation, calming the mind and body and putting them into a state that allows sleep. They also divert attention away from the distractions that may be preventing sleep, such as an overactive mind, worry, or pain.

Relaxation techniques work very well for many people. Others become anxious about what will happen if the technique doesn't work, or when the tape finishes or the exercise stops.

Goal
To fall asleep quickly and effectively at least seven nights out of every 10.

Action
- If you're having difficulty getting to sleep because your mind is too active or your body is too restless, try a relaxation technique.
- Drawing on your experience of what has been helpful in the past, choose one of the following:
  - Something that creates a relaxing environment, such as an audiotape with natural noises. Use a tape player that will automatically stop at the end of the tape, so that you don't have to worry about staying awake to switch it off
  - A technique that focuses on your body, such as progressive relaxation of your muscles ('Feel your toes. Tighten the muscles then release and relax them. Make them as loose as you can. Now feel the soles of your feet … ')
  - Something that relaxes your mind, like a visualization technique ('Imagine you're on a tropical beach … ')
- Persist with the technique for at least two weeks. Such techniques will work much better if they're used in conjunction with the 'Twenty-one nights to better sleep' programme

Worry anticipation
This is a useful technique for reducing the problems associated with an overactive brain when you're trying to get to sleep, especially if you're also likely to worry.

Goal
To have at least seven nights out of every 10 unbothered by worry or stress.

Action
- Set aside 20 to 30 minutes in the late afternoon or early evening

(but more than two hours before bedtime) to think quietly about everything that's worrying you.

- Imagine the worst possible outcomes. Don't leave all those 'what-ifs' for the middle of the night!
- Put your problems in some kind of order. In the last half of your session, focus on the one or two problems that appear to be the most serious or the most pressing.
- Decide on one or two things that you can actually do, even if those things might only solve a small part of the problem, or even if you can't see exactly how they would be helpful. For example, you might want to let someone know how you feel about something, talk to a confidant such as an old friend or spiritual guide, or plan something to take your mind off a situation.
- If the basic problem is one of confrontation, seek first to evaluate your position, preferably with the help of someone who isn't emotionally involved in this particular problem. Next, think about the point of view of the person who is causing the trouble. Again, you might want to enlist the help of a third party.
- If you wake up in the night and start to worry, refer back to your evening's session and especially to the actions that you intend to take.

Nasal CPAP (Continuous positive airway pressure)
This is a device prescribed by a sleep specialist or doctor that blows room air through your nose as you sleep. The pressure of the air keeps the upper airway open, preventing breathing problems in your sleep.

Goal
If this device has been prescribed for you for a breathing problem, you should use it whenever you're asleep. It should be comfortable and make you feel better when you're awake.

Action
- Follow the advice of your CPAP supplier.
- Remember that the masks and tubing become less flexible and more prone to leak with age. They'll probably need to be replaced every 12 to 18 months.
- Even if CPAP is successful, do as much as you can to improve your

health and reduce the severity of your breathing problems.

- See your doctor if:
  - you no longer wear the CPAP for all the time that you are asleep, either intentionally or because you awaken and find that you have pulled it off, and the suggestions given here are not helpful
  - it's been more than a year or two since you last saw your doctor CPAP equipment and supplies are improving all the time and you may be able to benefit from some of these improvements
  - you've started to snore or have pauses in your breathing again Even mild snoring may indicate an inadequate pressure
  - you've begun to experience unwelcome sleepiness

Weight management

Fatty tissue and sheer body mass can make the breathing problems of your sleep worse, but unfortunately, reversing weight gain is not a simple or guaranteed solution to those problems. Only about 20 per cent of sleep patients successfully maintain their weight loss over a two-year period. However, the distribution of fatty tissue is more important than your overall weight.

Goal

To minimize the impact of being overweight on your sleep.

Action

- Focus on a healthy, enjoyable, balanced lifestyle, not just on your weight.
- Avoid crash diets unless recommended for medical reasons. In general, try to lose no more than a pound or two a week.
- The most successful forms of weight management involve eating less fatty foods, eating more fruits and vegetables so that you do not feel hungry, and obtaining adequate exercise that's appropriate for your general health.
- See your doctor if:
  - weight gain, or loss, is relatively sudden
  - weight gain is the result of swelling, for example of your legs or ankles
  - you also have difficulty breathing